# Depression in Marriage

TREATMENT MANUALS FOR PRACTITIONERS
David H. Barlow, *Editor*


DEPRESSION IN MARRIAGE
A MODEL FOR ETIOLOGY AND TREATMENT
Steven R. H. Beach, Evelyn E. Sandeen,
and K. Daniel O'Leary

TREATING ALCOHOL DEPENDENCE
A COPING SKILLS TRAINING GUIDE
Peter M. Monti, David B. Abrams,
Ronald M. Kadden, and Ned L. Cooney

SELF-MANAGEMENT FOR ADOLESCENTS
A SKILLS-TRAINING PROGRAM
MANAGING EVERYDAY PROBLEMS
Thomas A. Brigham

PSYCHOLOGICAL TREATMENT OF PANIC
David H. Barlow and Jerome A. Cerny

# Depression in Marriage
## A Model for Etiology and Treatment

STEVEN R. H. BEACH
University of Georgia

EVELYN E. SANDEEN
K. DANIEL O'LEARY
State University of New York at Stony Brook

*Editor's Note by David H. Barlow*
*Foreword by Robert L. Weiss*

THE GUILFORD PRESS
New York   London

© 1990 The Guilford Press
A Division of Guilford Publications, Inc.
72 Spring Street, New York, NY 10012

Printed in the United States of America

This book is printed on acid-free paper

Last digit is print number: 9 8 7 6 5 4 3 2 1

Library of Congress Cataloging-in-Publication Data

Beach, Steven R. H.
    Depression in marriage: a model for etiology and treatment /
Steven R. H. Beach, Evelyn E. Sandeen, K. Daniel O'Leary; editor's
note by David H. Barlow; foreword by Robert L. Weiss.
        p.   cm.—(Treatment manuals for practitioners)
    Includes bibliographical references.
    ISBN 0-89862-205-0.—ISBN 0-89862-216-6 (pbk.)
    1. Marital psychotherapy.   2. Depression, Mental—Treatment.
3. Depression, Mental—Etiology.   I. Sandeen, Evelyn.   II. O'Leary,
K. Daniel, 1940–     .   III. Barlow, David H.   IV. Title. V. Series.
    [DNLM: 1. Depression—etiology.   2. Depression—therapy.
3. Marital Therapy.   WM 171 B365d]
    RC488.5.B379   1990
    616.89'156—dc20
    DNLM/DLC
for Library of Congress                                     90-2775
                                                               CIP

# Editor's Note

Few disorders have as much of an impact on interpersonal relations as does depression. Evidence suggests that 50% of depressed women experience marital difficulties and that 50% of women with marital problems are depressed. The implication of these findings is that it is very difficult, if not impossible, to treat one without considering the other in the majority of cases. Now, Beach, Sandeen, and O'Leary present for the first time their program for treating depression in a marital context. Even therapists who are well-seasoned veterans in treating either depression or marital discord will want to be aware of these exciting new advances in assessment and treatment. Supported by many years of research, this program is perhaps the finest example of recent trends to integrate the techniques emanating from cognitive-behavioral approaches with the insights of interpersonal systems theory. Psychopathology never occurs in a vacuum, and the intertwining of depression and marital problems is perhaps the most visible example of this truism. My own reading of this superb manual suggests that therapists treating other psychopathology will benefit from reading how techniques can be integrated successfully into a dysfunctional interpersonal system. Since every treatment ultimately will have to be so integrated, this model is sure to become increasingly important.

David H. Barlow
*State University of New York at Albany*

# Foreword

*"All things extreme, regress to the mean."*

When behavioral marital therapy first came upon the scene in the late 1960s and early '70s, it was often difficult to see the rider for the glare of the knight's shining armor. It was extreme, in arrogance, technique, and promise. If there is one thing to characterize the development of BMT, now as we enter a new decade—approaching our escape velocity for the century itself—it is a palpable reduction in *hubris*. Gone are the ritualistic chants for standardization, imploring everyone to do "it" in the fashion prescribed by the BMT protocol. After many decades and thousands of practitioner hours spent in all forms of therapy, is there perhaps (as Jerome Frank has suggested) a common mass of therapy lore that cuts across the different theoretical persuasions? Research has shown that just about any therapy is consistently better than no-therapy controls. Some have taken this to also mean that all therapies operate from a common base and that they are not—indeed should not be—differentially effective. For others this conclusion may be too much a regression to the mean.

In this clinical manual, Beach, Sandeen, and O'Leary display an acceptable instance of the regression-to-the-mean effect. It is seriously different from others of its genre purporting to teach the complexities of clinical marital therapy skills. I sense a conscious recognition by clinical researchers and publishers alike that practitioners are not consumers of research reports, even though the quantity and, gladly in many cases, the quality has risen enormously. These authors have attempted, and in my view succeeded admirably, to retain some very important attitudes characteristic of the early BMT ethos while also recognizing that no single manualized approach is going to meet all therapy circumstances. They do this by building skillfully on the empirical tradition that has characterized BMT and combining it with developments in our understanding of affective disorders. If depression is important to marital quality then it behooves us to know something about depression, and not to view it as an annoying epiphenomenon. Inevitably as marital therapists we must acknowledge depression as part of the total relationship. Regardless of who is depressed the relationship must deal with it. While maintaining an allegiance to research the authors are conspicuous in their willingness to tap what I suspect is some of the more common therapy lore.

The tone of this manual is different also. When there are no empirical data to support this or that intervention technique the authors make it quite clear that they are drawing upon their clinical experiences with depression in marriage. This allows the reader to compare his or her experience with the authors' view of the unicorn. That should prove very helpful to the conscientious practitioner who has attempted to divine useful techniques, often analogues, buried in the fine print of the "Procedures" sections of otherwise promising journal papers.

This manual explicitly recognizes that marriage may eventually prove to be a micro-model for understanding the larger context of psychosocial adjustment—for example, viewing the role of marital distress in health issues. Depression is indeed the common cold of psychopathology; but so is the struggle so many of the 90+% of us who ever get married engage in to find an acceptable accommodation to a chosen other. The book takes a giant step beyond the eclectic fare I am familiar with: Beach et al. argue for a *systematic* approach in conceptualizing marital therapy. They carefully walk the fine line between "Manual, manual on the wall, who is the most correct of all?" and what is often conceptual anarchy on the other hand.

Is this to become an era of still other manuals produced in the format of "*X* in Marriage," where *X* can be any other notable psychological disorder? That is certainly a risk to be faced in the current upwelling of practitioner manuals. But there is one thing I believe we have learned from BMT: The applicability of our intervention techniques is widespread. The problem is getting the clients to use them! Finding a consumer-friendly vehicle for increasing positives is really at issue. Certainly in the face of a serious depression one is not going to ask enthusiastically, "And just what do *you* two do for fun?" But there are techniques available. Even with what may already have become an uncritical acceptance of cognitive techniques, there are issues of technique acceptability that need to be addressed; these authors take the beginning steps to do so. They are on the right track when they acknowledge that there is a need for distinctly marriage-focused cognitive interventions, and not just warmed-over techniques from individual therapies.

I was particularly impressed to read the authors' sound advice that marital therapy may not be the intervention of choice in all cases. Marital therapy based on BMT, as this model is, needs to recognize that it is not a universal marital lubricant. Whether the systems people know something that we don't is yet to be determined—they seem to work with any and all problems! I strongly agree with the present authors that our up-front assessment should answer the question, "Is this a marital problem amenable to what we can do technique-wise?" Just saying "no," after all, *may* be the socially responsible thing to do.

Their topic is socially important, and the authors treatment of it scholarly and clinically relevant. If this be a regression to the mean it will be one very useful to the many who struggle daily with discordant, depressive marriages.

Robert L. Weiss
*Oregon Marital Studies Program*

# Preface

This book describes the theoretical and empirical foundations of marital intervention with depressed patients. The interventions we detail represent an alternative or adjunct to individual and somatic interventions for depression. We have found the marital approach to be especially effective in alleviating depression in women who are both depressed and maritally discordant. Ignored, a discordant marital environment may overwhelm biological or individually oriented treatments of depression. Properly utilized, however, marital therapy may alleviate depressive symptomatology.

Biological, individual, and marital treatments all have a valid place in the treatment of depression. Throughout the book we provide guidelines for determining when marital therapy for depression is the best choice, when it should be used as an adjunct to other forms of therapy, and when it is not the treatment of choice.

The book consists of two sections. In Section I we present information about depression. We believe it is virtually impossible to work effectively with depressed patients in discordant marriages without a clear understanding of the symptoms of depression, the pathways leading to depression, and the role of marriage in the etiology and maintenance of depression. Therefore, we first describe various types of depression and present information on the etiologies of depression. We then introduce the marital discord model of depression, which provides the structure for the interventions discussed later.

In Section II we outline a marital treatment for co-occurring depression and marital discord. We divide therapy into three stages: (1) the initial stage, which focuses on the elimination of severe stressors and the enhancement of marital cohesion and self-esteem support; (2) the middle stage, which focuses on restructuring a variety of dysfunctional interaction patterns; and (3) the termination stage, which focuses on disengaging from therapy in a way that promotes optimal maintenance of both marital satisfaction and improved mood. Finally, we discuss our own outcome work and related empirical evaluations of the effectiveness of marital therapy in the treatment of depression. The treatment research is especially exciting because marital therapy can be a very viable treatment not only for marital discord but for depression as well.

We gratefully acknowledge the National Institute of Mental Health funding that has allowed us to focus our attention on the use of marital therapy in the treatment of depression and has facilitated greatly the development of this book. In particular, NIMH Grant Nos. MH38390 and MH42085 directly supported our work. We also thank those who have participated in our research efforts as assistants, therapists, and patients. Permission to use therapy material in our research was essential. However, no individuals are named or identified in any of the case material included in the book. Where necessary, changes were made in case descriptions to ensure anonymity of all participants.

Steven R. H. Beach
Evelyn E. Sandeen
K. Daniel O'Leary

# Contents

# Contents

# I

# UNDERSTANDING CO-OCCURRING DEPRESSION AND MARITAL DISCORD

# 1

## Depression: The Basic Facts

### Why Should I Learn about Depression?

Many good marital therapists may wonder why they should update their knowledge about depression before attempting to work with a depressed and maritally discordant population. Why should good marital therapists who are going to treat married people using a *marital* intervention take time to learn or to review basic information about diagnosis, prevalence, etiology, and alternative approaches to the treatment of depression? Because of such thoughts, some practitioners may have ignored important developments in the fast-paced field of depression research. Nevertheless, a thorough grounding in the basics of depression should be considered a prerequisite to conducting marital therapy with a depressed population. Diagnostic issues are becoming more relevant to providing the most effective treatments. Dealing with suicide and making choices about the use of individual or marital therapy are tricky issues that require a broad knowledge base about the depressive disorders. Knowing how to differentiate unipolar and bipolar depression requires more than simple descriptions of symptomatology. Knowing when to refer a patient for medication or adjunctive medical treatment is becoming more and more important. Misinterpretation of depressive symptoms can lead to the imparting of erroneous information in the course of marital therapy. Clinicians should know when symptoms resemble depression but are reflections of medical or other psychological disorders. Further, in providing treatment today, all professionals should know about the major alternative forms of treatment and their efficacy in helping clients, and they should help patients make rational choices about the course of therapy they wish to pursue. Accordingly, a thorough knowledge of the basic facts about depression is critical for marital and family therapists who will be assessing and/or treating this population.

## Why Should I Learn about Marital Discord?

A similar question may occur to the clinician who is already well versed in one of the empirically documented individual approaches for the treatment of depression. Why should the clinician who already knows how to implement an effective individual approach to depression learn about marital approaches to treatment for depressed clients who happen to be maritally discordant as well? Again, we believe such thoughts do occur to practicing therapists and may lead them to ignore developments in the field of marital therapy when treating depression. Unfortunately, any clinician treating depressed individuals will see many depressed people with serious marital discord. In fact, approximately 50% of depressed women are maritally discordant (Rounsaville, Weissman, Prusoff, & Herceg-Baron, 1979a, 1979b) and approximately 50% of maritally discordant women are depressed (Beach, Jouriles, & O'Leary, 1985; Weissman, 1987). Of course, some people develop depression who are not maritally discordant and who have no significant relationship problems. People become depressed for varied reasons, such as losing their jobs or becoming ill. What we wish to emphasize here, however, is that marital discord is both a cause and a correlate of depression in a large number of individuals. We will develop a model in this book documenting the link between marital discord and depression, and we hope that any clinician or researcher who treats depressed individuals will be convinced that knowledge of the role of marital problems in the development and maintenance of depression is critical for understanding and treating their patients.

## Why Should I Learn about Marital Therapy for Depression?

Marital therapy with depressed persons is not simply standard marital therapy as practiced with the general marital therapy client; neither is marital therapy with depressed persons simply applying an individual treatment of depression (e.g., cognitive-behavior therapy) in a couples' context. Marital therapy for the treatment of depression as presented in this book is a hybrid therapy that utilizes a marital discord model of depression. Armed with information about both depression and marital discord, therapists will be able to use our theoretical model to provide interventions that will fit very reasonably with the views that these depressed people have about their problems. Moreover, the use of our model will aid clinicians in processing both diagnostic and treatment information and in tailoring the treatment procedures to needs of depressed people in a fashion that maximizes the likelihood of success.

This chapter is designed as a review of the literature on diagnosis, prevalence, incidence, and risk factors associated with depression. Further, it provides information about the differential diagnosis of types of depression. This information is designed to supplement basic graduate training in psychopathology, and some previous clinical supervision is expected. For those who wish to investigate primary sources, references are liberally cited.

## General Definition

Almost everyone gets down in the dumps or has the blues sometimes. Feeling sad or dejected is clearly a normal part of the spectrum of human emotion. This situation is so common that a very important issue is how to separate a normal "blue" or "down" mood or emotion from an abnormal clinical state. As we shall soon see, most clinicians use measures of intensity, severity, and duration of these emotions to separate the almost unavoidable human experience of sadness and dejection from clinical depression.

Depression is seen in all social classes, races, and ethnic groups. It is so pervasive that it has been called "the common cold of mental illness" in the popular press (Gelman, 1987). It is approximately twice as common among women as it is among men. Depression is seen among all occupations, but it is most common among people in the arts and humanities. Famous individuals such as Abraham Lincoln and Winston Churchill who coped with depression were afflicted with what Churchill called "the black dog." More recently, Senator Thomas Eagleton and astronaut Edwin Aldrin were known to have bouts of serious depression.

The specific defining features of depressive disorders (major depression and dysthymia) and bipolar disorders (bipolar disorder and cyclothymia) as presented in the third, revised edition of the *Diagnostic and Statistical Manual of Mental Disorders* (DSM-III-R; American Psychiatric Association, 1987) are presented in Table 1-1.

## Prevalence and Incidence

Of all problems that are mentioned by patients at psychological and psychiatric clinics, some form of depression is most common. It is estimated that approximately 25% of women in the United States will experience at least one significant depression during their lives (Boyd & Klerman, 1978). Contrary to a popular misconception that depression is most common among the elderly, it is actually most common in 25- to

TABLE 1-1. Subclassification of Mood Disorders and Diagnostic Criteria

Mood disorders are divided into depressive disorders and bipolar disorders, and in turn there are two subclassifications of each of these disorders.

## I. Depressive disorders

A. *Major depression.* Major depression involves one or more major depressive episodes. A major depressive episode must meet the following criteria:

1. At least five of the following symptoms have been present during the same 2-week period and represent a change from previous functioning; at least one of the symptoms is either (a) depressed mood, or (b) loss of interest or pleasure. (Do not include symptoms that are clearly due to a physical condition, mood-incongruent delusions or hallucinations, incoherence, or marked loosening of associations.)

   (a) depressed mood (or can be irritable mood in children and adolescents) most of the day, nearly every day, as indicated either by subjective account or observation by others

   (b) markedly diminished interest or pleasure in all, or almost all, activities most of the day, nearly every day (as indicated either by subjective account or observation by others of apathy most of the time)

   (c) significant weight loss or weight gain when not dieting (e.g., more than 5% of body weight in a month), or decrease or increase in appetite nearly every day (in children, consider failure to make expected weight gains)

   (d) insomnia or hypersomnia nearly every day

   (e) psychomotor agitation or retardation nearly every day (observable by others, not merely subjective feelings of restlessness or being slowed down)

   (f) fatigue or loss of energy nearly every day

   (g) feelings of worthlessness or excessive or inappropriate guilt (which may be delusional) nearly every day (not merely self-reproach or guilt about being sick)

   (h) diminished ability to think or concentrate, or indecisiveness, nearly every day (either by subjective account or as observed by others)

   (i) recurrent thoughts of death (not just fear of dying), recurrent suicidal ideation without a specific plan, or a suicide attempt or a specific plan for committing suicide

2. (a) It cannot be established that an organic factor initiated and maintained the disturbance.

   (b) The disturbance is not a normal reaction to the death of a loved one (uncomplicated bereavement).

   *Note*: Morbid preoccupation with worthlessness, suicidal ideation, marked functional impairment or psychomotor retardation, or prolonged duration suggest bereavement complicated by major depression.

3. At no time during the disturbance have there been delusions or hallucinations for as long as 2 weeks in the absence of prominent mood symptoms (i.e., before the mood symptoms developed or after they have remitted).

4. Not superimposed on schizophrenia, schizophreniform disorder, delusional disorder, or psychotic disorder NOS.

*(continued)*

TABLE 1-1. (Continued)

B. *Dysthymia.*
1. Depressed mood (or can be irritable mood in children and adolescents) for most of the day, more days than not, as indicated either by subjective account or observation by others, for at least 2 years (1 year for children and adolescents)
2. Presence, while depressed, of at least two of the following:
    (a) poor appetite or overeating
    (b) insomnia or hypersomnia
    (c) low energy or fatigue
    (d) low self-esteem
    (e) poor concentration or difficulty making decisions
    (f) feelings of hopelessness
3. During a 2-year period (1-year for children and adolescents) of the disturbance, never without the symptoms in 1 for more than 2 months at a time.
4. No evidence of an unequivocal major depressive episode during the first 2 years (1 year for children and adolescents) of the disturbance.

## II. Bipolar disorders

A. *Bipolar disorder.* A bipolar disorder involves one or more manic episodes (usually with one or more major depressive episodes). A manic episode must meet the following criteria:
*Note*: A hypomanic is defined as meeting criteria 1 and 2, but not 3, that is, no marked impairment.
1. A distinct period of abnormally and persistently elevated, expansive, or irritable mood.
2. During the period of mood disturbance, at least three of the following symptoms have persisted (four if the mood is only irritable) and have been present to a significant degree:
    (a) inflated self-esteem or grandiosity
    (b) decreased need for sleep (e.g., feels rested after only 3 hours of sleep)
    (c) more talkative than usual or pressure to keep talking
    (d) flight of ideas or subjective experience that thoughts are racing
    (e) distractibility (i.e., attention too easily drawn to unimportant or irrelevant external stimuli)
    (f) increase in goal-directed activity (either socially, at work or school, or sexually) or psychomotor agitation
    (g) excessive involvement in pleasurable activities that have a high potential for painful consequences (e.g., the person engages in unrestrained buying sprees, sexual indiscretions, or foolish business investments)
3. Mood disturbance sufficiently severe to cause marked impairment in occupational functioning or in usual social activities or relationships with others, or to necessitate hospitalization to prevent harm to self or others.
4. At no time during the disturbance have there been delusions or hallucinations for as long as 2 weeks in the absence of prominent mood symptoms (i.e., before the mood symptoms developed or after they have remitted).

(continued)

---

**TABLE 1-1.** (Continued)

---

5. Not superimposed on schizophrenia, schizophreniform disorder, delusional disorder, or psychotic disorder NOS.
6. It cannot be established that an organic factor initiated and maintained the disturbance.

B. *Cyclothymia.* Cyclothymia involves numerous hypomanic episode periods alternating with depressive symptoms. To be diagnosed cyclothymic, a patient must meet the following criteria:

1. For at least 2 years (1 year for children and adolescents), presence of numerous hypomanic episodes and numerous periods with depressed mood or loss of interest or pleasure that did not meet criterion 1 of major depressive episode.
2. During a 2-year period (1-year in children and adolescents) of the disturbance, never without hypomanic or depressive symptoms for more than 2 months at a time.
3. No clear evidence of a major depressive episode or manic episode during the first 2 years of the disturbance (or 1 year in children and adolescents).
   *Note*: After this minimum period of cyclothymia, there may be superimposed manic or major depressive episodes, in which case the additional diagnosis of bipolar disorder or bipolar disorder NOS should be given.
4. Not superimposed on a chronic psychotic disorder, such as schizophrenia or delusional disorder.
5. It cannot be established that an organic factor initiated and maintained the disturbance (e.g., repeated intoxication from drugs or alcohol).

---

*Note.* From American Psychiatric Association. (1987). *Diagnostic and statistical manual of mental disorders* (3rd ed.—rev.), pp. 217, 222–223, 227–228, 232. Washington, DC: Author. Copyright 1987 by the American Psychiatric Association. Adapted by permission.

44-year-olds (Robins et al., 1984). About 10% of the college population report moderate depression, and 5% report severe depression (Craighead, Kennedy, Raczynski, & Dow, 1984). Women experience depression approximately twice as frequently as men (Nolen-Hoeksema, 1987), and this sex difference exists across diverse cultures and countries throughout the world, with exceptions in developing countries and among the elderly. About 6% of women are hospitalized at some point for depression, while only 3% of men are (American Psychiatric Association, 1980).

When one examines the prevalence or percentage of a population who have had specific subtypes of affective disorders such as the depressive disorders or the bipolar disorders, the figures as reflected in DSM-III-R (American Psychiatric Association, 1987) are as indicated below.

*Major Depression.* While prevalence figures vary considerably, it appears that approximately 9% to 26% of women and 5% to 12% of men have had a major depressive disorder at one time in their lives. Examination of populations to determine who currently has the disorder indicate that about 7% to 8% of women and 3% of men have it.

*Dysthymia.* There are not enough studies about this problem to allow precise prevalence or incidence figures to be given, and the boundaries of major depression and dysthymia are unclear, especially in children. Among adults the disorder is apparently more common in females, but in children it appears to occur equally in both sexes.

*Bipolar Disorders.* It is estimated that approximately 0.5% to 1% of the population have had this disorder, and it appears with equal rates in men and women (unlike major depression).

*Cyclothymia.* It is estimated that 0.5% to 3% of the population have had this problem at least once in their lives, and the problem is equally common in men and women.

Largely because the prevalence of unipolar depression is much greater than that of bipolar depression, most of the research on depression, especially psychological research, has been about major depression. We too shall discuss the etiology and treatment of major depression, since our treatment, which will be outlined later, was designed for persons experiencing major depression. While bipolar disorders are very intriguing, they are seen by most researchers as having a much stronger genetic component than unipolar disorders. This stronger genetic influence may be responsible for the general belief that bipolar depressives are less responsive to psychological therapies than are unipolar depressives. In practice, however, it should be recognized that the distinction between unipolar and bipolar disorders is not always clear, particularly the distinction between the unipolar depressive and the depressive phase of a bipolar disorder. Consequently, it should be apparent that knowing the psychological history of an individual is very important in making this distinction and that the use of psychological tests that focus on a person's affective state at a particular point can be misleading in making a diagnosis without a carefully honed assessment interview. In addition, assessing for information about family history of psychopathology may be helpful in identifying some depressives who might best be considered under the bipolar spectrum.

## Symptoms of Major Depression

The most prominent affective symptom in major depression is dysphoric mood. The term *dysphoria* is derived from the Greek words *dys* (hard) and *pherein* (to bear), and dysphoria refers to a generalized feeling of lack of well-being, especially an abnormal feeling of discontent, anxiety, or physical discomfort. As reflected in this definition, feelings of anxiousness and fearfulness are often seen in major depression. As Hamilton (1982) noted, the three most common symptoms seen in depression are depressed mood, loss of interest, and anxiety. He reported that difficulty falling asleep, loss of appetite, lack of energy and easy fatigue, and suicidal thoughts come next in order of frequency. In an interesting discussion of symptom presentation, Hamilton indicated that less educated or psychologically sophisticated patients tend to emphasize physical symptoms and underplay their feelings of depression and anxiety. Upon questioning, however, they will admit to a feeling of "flatness" or "loss of feeling." At the outset of major depression, individuals will often weep and cry for no apparent reason. After several months, they may report that they feel like crying but it no longer seems feasible. They will avoid company and group activities, though the depression may not be apparent to many outsiders. Consequently, interviews with spouses or relatives are very important.

Loss of interest is reflected in the cessation or marked diminution of hobbies or lack of interest in work. At work, decision making may become labored and avoided more and more. Actual activities often involve work that reflects avoidance of the important tasks at hand; cleaning and filing may occupy a large portion of the individual's time.

Anxiety is seen in tenseness and in the inability to relax. Patients often complain of symptoms of anxiety, such as palpitations and sweating.

Delay in getting to sleep is the most common form of sleep disturbance. While trying to get to sleep, the depressed person worries and ruminates about events of the day. Lower sleep efficiency and more awake time during the night characterize depressed adolescents, though their REM sleep is not different from that of control subjects (Goetz et al., 1987). Sad dreams are common if any dreams are reported.

Suicidal thoughts are common in depressive clients, and in long-term follow-up it has been found that approximately 15% of depressed individuals eventually kill themselves. Alternatively viewed, however, approximately 60% of suicides are believed to be caused by depression or depression in association with alcohol abuse. As has been vividly portrayed in the media, teenage suicide in the United States is increasing at an alarming rate (Peck, 1989). It is important to assess for this problem in all cases of depression. The threat of suicide becomes greater as evidence accumulates for the therapist that the patient or client has made such attempts in the past or has made clear plans to do so in the future. As Schneidman, Farberow, and Litman (1970) showed, approximately 80% of suicides have a recognizable presuicidal phase. Any therapist who sees depressed clients should be sensitive to issues regarding this fatal outcome associated with depression.

## Conditions Associated with Major Depressive Disorder

The most common problem associated with depression is anxiety. In fact, scales of depression and anxiety often correlate at approximately 0.60 (Beck, Brown, Steer, Eidelson, & Riskind, 1987). Since the correlation between these variables is so high, it has led some to question whether depression and anxiety are discrete disorders or are part of the same disorder. Beck (1976) has argued that the cognitive model of psychopathology stipulates that each neurotic disorder can be characterized by a cognitive content specific to that disorder. He holds that the automatic thoughts of the depressed person center around the theme of self-deprecation and negative attitudes toward the world and the future. On the other hand, he holds that individuals with anxiety disorders, characterized by the theme of danger, tend to misread their experiences as "constituting either a physical or psychosocial threat and to overestimate both the probability and intensity of anticipated harm in future situations" (Beck et al., 1987, p. 179). Beck and colleagues have developed the Cognitive Checklist, which enables one to differentiate the thoughts relevant to anxiety and depression. Further, using a structured clinical interview, major depressive disorders and generalized anxiety disorders can be reliably diagnosed (kappas for each are, respectively, .72 and .79; Riskind, Beck, Berchick, Brown, & Steer, 1987).

Alcohol abuse is commonly associated with depression. According to Vaillant (1988), alcoholism is by far a more common cause of depression than depression is of alcoholism. Therefore, in treating an alcoholic who is depressed, a cessation in drinking may lead to a reduction of depressive symptomatology.

Endocrine abnormalities such as hyperthyroidism and hypothyroidism are often associated with depressive symptoms. Some forms of cancer, some types of stroke, and some forms of degenerative disease have associated depressive symptomatology. These conditions are sometimes difficult to distinguish from depression not caused by an organic problem. Therefore, it is always important to be alert to possible signs of organic involvement both in the assessment phase and in treatment situations where little progress is being made, since the continued depression may be due to organic problems. Clinicians should also be aware that there are sources containing information about certain physical conditions (such as brain dysfunction) that mimic psychological conditions such as depression (cf. Berg, Franzen, & Wedding, 1987, for brain dysfunction, and Cameron, 1987, for medical conditions associated with depression). Further, if a clinician suspects that a medical condition may be producing the depression, a referral for diagnostic medical evaluation or a second opinion is certainly in order.

Table 1-2 (from Hales, 1986) summarizes the medications and medical conditions associated with depressive symptoms. We will simply
review some of the most common medications and conditions associated
with depression. The clinician who suspects that any of the medications
or medical conditions may be causing depression in a particular case
should consult Hales (1986) for further details.

Several antihypertensive medications may cause depressive symptoms. For example, as many as 10% of cases receiving methyldopa
experienced depressive symptoms, and reserpine may be associated with
depression, especially in those cases with a family background of depression. Propranolol and other beta-blockers may cause depressive symptoms in as many as 30% of the cases.

Depressive symptoms are often observed in patients receiving steroid
treatments. Cancer patients receiving steroids as part of their chemother-
apy regimen are especially at risk for developing depressive symptoms.

---

TABLE 1-2. Medications and Medical Conditions Associated with Depressive Symptoms

---

*Medications*
  Anti-anxiety agents, carbidopa, clonidine, corticosteroids, digitalis, ethambutol, guane-
  thidine, indomethacin, levodopa, methyldopa, oral contraceptives, reserpine, propranolol, sedative-hypnotics

*Medical conditions*
  Cardiovascular
    Myocardial infarction
  Collagen
    Systemic lupus erythematosus
  Drug withdrawal states
    Amphetamines, cocaine
  Endocrine
    Addison disease, Cushing syndrome, diabetes mellitus, hyperparathyroidism, hyper-
    thyroidism, hypothyroidism
  Infectious
    Hepatitis, influenza, mononucleosis, tuberculosis
  Malignant
    Pancreatic carcinoma
  Metabolic
    Multiple sclerosis, Parkinson disease, Wilson disease, seizure disorders, stroke
  Nutritional
    B12, B6, folic acid, thiamine

---

*Note.* From Hales, R. E. (1986). The diagnosis and treatment of psychiatric disorders in medically ill
patients. *Military Medicine, 151,* 592. Copyright 1986 by the Association of Military Surgeons of the
U.S. Reprinted by permission of the publisher and author.

Finally, patients with Parkinson disease treated with levodopa may experience depression associated with the medication use. Therapists should always inquire about whether their client or patient is taking any medication, since treatment for depression in the absence of referral for medical consultation, when the depression potentially has been caused by medication, would be foolish.

## Bereavement

As noted by Clayton (1982), bereavement is a universal human condition. In fact, the death of a loved one is one of the most traumatic experiences we ever face. Since bereavement is a universal human condition, it is important to know how long most people experience the symptoms usually associated with it. Using widowers as a sample of interest, Clayton found that more than one-third of all widowers were still experiencing crying, sleep disturbance, low mood, and restlessness 13 months following the death of their spouses.

Interestingly, Blanchard, Blanchard, and Becker (1976) in a retrospective study of widows found that as the physiological symptoms of depression abate, psychological symptoms such as hopelessness and feeling angry become more prominent. Since bereaved individuals have symptoms of depression, a logical question is what percentage of these individuals would meet diagnostic criteria for depression. With widows of average age 62, Clayton, Halikas, and Maurice (1982) found 35% at 1 month, 25% at 4 months, and 17% at 1 year would be classified as depressed. Of special interest, except for those already ill, Clayton (1982) reported that longitudinal studies indicate that older men and women have very few changes in their physical health, visits to physicians, and hospitalizations after bereavement. On the other hand, all studies report an increase in alcohol use, cigarette smoking, and tranquilizers or hypnotics. Finally, there is no increase in mortality for women following the death of a spouse, but there is an increased mortality risk for men in the first 6 months of bereavement. Interestingly, in contrast to those with major depressive disorders, suicidal thoughts are uncommon (affecting less than 10% of the population) in the bereaved.

A final question of critical interest to the clinician is what, if anything, should be done for the bereaved patient. There have been no controlled studies on the treatment of the bereaved, but it has been found in retrospective studies of bereaved individuals that reviewing the terminal illness or last few months of a partner's life are seen as beneficial by the bereaved. The general belief is that bereaved individuals should only receive treatment if the symptoms persist and if they are quite prominent.

Otherwise, simple support from family and friends, along with the passage of time, is enough to alleviate the dysphoria.

## Depression Associated with Organic Disorders and Psychotic Features

The diagnosis of major depressive disorder is made only when it cannot be established that an organic factor caused or is maintaining the depression. If an individual has both a cancerous condition and depressed mood and if the depression could be attributed to organic changes resulting from the cancer, the depression would be considered an organic mood disorder rather than a major depressive episode. While not frequent in outpatient practices, organic causes of depressed mood should not be arbitrarily ruled out. Interventions targeted at improving the marital relationship are unlikely to be sufficient to reduce depressed mood due to organic factors.

Schizophrenics often have dysphoric mood that is intermittently mixed with anger and anxiety. The dysphoric mood would not necessarily be seen in our model as a function of marital discord. However, schizophrenics in remission are more likely to be rehospitalized if their significant others (parents or spouses) are critical of them (cf. Goldstein, 1985). Consequently, while we certainly do not view the causes of schizophrenia as family or marital discord (O'Leary & Wilson, 1987), it is certainly possible that marital or family problems can play a role in triggering a psychotic episode and/or rehospitalization.

Further, the model of marital discord and depression presented in this book may in fact be able to be applied to psychological and psychiatric conditions other than unipolar depression. For example, marital discord may indeed be a potent enough stressor to lead individuals to have a psychotic episode associated with bipolar depression. Marital discord and spouse abuse are certainly associated with suicide attempts (Welz, 1988), and marital discord is clearly a precipitant of drinking binges in individuals prone to alcohol abuse (Marlatt & Gordon, 1985). Thus, while we are not arguing that marital discord be seen as a cause of organic or psychotic features of various psychiatric problems, we are emphasizing that marital problems may be very potent stressors that can trigger individuals to enter states or engage in behaviors that will lead them to have psychotic and/or organic features. Finally, we have seen improvements in the moods of individuals with a history of schizophrenic episodes or bouts of alcoholism, and it is clear that therapy following from the marital model of depression potentially can play a useful role in supplementing pharmacological treatment and involvement in Alcoholics Anonymous, respectively, in these cases.

## Demographic Risk Factors for Depression

## Gender

In almost all industrialized countries, depression occurs in women about twice as often as in men (Nolen-Hoeksema, 1987; Weissman, 1987). Interestingly, the different rates of depression for men and women are not found in developing countries, such as India, Iraq, New Guinea, and Zimbabwe. Many people, on hearing about the greater rates of depression in women than men, respond that this may be due simply to women's greater likelihood of seeking treatment for depression. Indeed, treatment for depression is more commonly sought by women, but when epidemiological studies are conducted among all residents of a community, more women than men are found to be depressed. In fact, community studies using a standard classification for diagnosis reveal about a 1.6 to 1.0 ratio of women to men with depression in the United States and elsewhere (Nolen-Hoeksema, 1987).

The explanation for the differential sex ratio is unclear (Boyd & Weissman, 1981; Wilson, O'Leary, & Nathan, in press). Two major sets of explanations have been proffered: biological explanations and psychological explanations. The major biological explanation to account for the sex difference in depression is hormonal. It has been theorized that the higher rates of depression in women are due to changes in progesterone and estrogen. Despite the attention that these explanations have received, they have not been confirmed. In fact, research on daily mood ratings and menstrual cycle have not revealed any systematic associations (e.g., Abplanap, Donnelly, & Rose, 1979). While it may be too early to discount this biological hypothesis altogether, there is little evidence to support this notion now.

The main psychological explanations used to explain the differential sex ratio finding are stress and coping styles. Though there have been studies linking stress and the severity of psychiatric symptoms, women do not report more stress than men. Further, when men and women are asked to report the stressful nature of life events, women do not perceive these events as more stressful than men (Uhlenhuth, Balter, Lipman, & Haberman, 1977; Uhlenhuth, Lipman, Balter, & Stern, 1974). A psychological explanation that has received increasing attention is the coping-style hypothesis. A number of reseachers have found that women respond differently from men to their own feelings of depression. Stated most simply, women tend to ruminate about the causes of their depressed mood, whereas men tend to engage in activities designed to distract themselves from their depressed mood (Nolen-Hoeksema, 1987).

## Age

The highest rate of nonbipolar depression is found in persons aged 18 to 44, with particularly high rates for women in this age range (Weissman, 1987). Incidence and prevalence rates appear to peak in the 35- to 45-year-old age range for women (Charney & Weissman, 1988). However, it now appears that age of onset for nonbipolar depression is decreasing.

## Cohort Effects

Any time that differences in depression or any other disorder are found to vary with age, it is necessary to ask whether a particular age group experienced some unusual stressors that would make them especially vulnerable to certain problems. This concern about levels of a disorder in a particular group is called a cohort effect.

　　While it appears that there has been some decrease in the prevalence of depression among older populations (over age 65), there appears to be a very clear increase in the rate of depression among younger populations. This finding appears to be true in both the United States and Europe. It seems that people born after 1945, the so-called baby-boom generation, are more likely to be depressed than those born before 1945. Further, using stratified random sampling of high school students in New York State, it has been found that self-reported rates of depression in adolescents are higher than the self-reported rates of depression in their parents (Kandel & Davies, 1982). In addition, depression appears to be more common in adolescents than in their parents in England (Rutter, Graham, Chadwick, & Yule, 1976). The reasons for the cohort effects are not yet clear, but it has been observed that rapidly increasing divorce rates and the increasing number of children born to single parents may be a contributing factor to the cohort effect. It is also possible that the increasing role of women in the workforce without a commensurate decrease in their role in the home may contribute to the increase in depression among younger populations. Further, as noted by Klerman (1988), the weakening of traditional psychosocial supports, such as the extended family and religious institutions, may also influence the increased rates of depression among young women.

## Marital Status

It has been alleged that men are bullish on marriage because it is good for them; similarly, it has been alleged that marriage is bad for women

(Bernard, 1972). In fact, when one looks at the overall rates of depression, they are highest in the unmarried and widowed groups. Further, the rates of depression for women are lowest among married women (Gove, Hughes, & Style, 1983). However, if the marriage is seen as unsatisfactory by the wife, the likelihood of her being depressed is as high as 50% (Beach et al., 1985; Weissman, 1985). In addition, a spouse in a discordant marriage appears to be 25 times more likely to be depressed than a spouse in a nondiscordant marriage, and this is true for both husbands and wives (Weissman, 1987). Further, as we will document later, there is increasing evidence to indicate that a discordant marriage leads to an increase in depressive symptomatology. Conversely, if a woman has an intimate with whom she can confide, such as a boyfriend or husband, this serves as a significant protection against depression (Brown & Harris, 1978).

## Social Class

Overall, some reviews indicate that no clear relation has been established between social class and unipolar depression (Boyd & Weissman, 1981). However, an epidemiological study conducted in the United States in the early 1980s indicated that being in the lower social classes is associated with higher levels of depressive symptoms (Hirschfeld & Cross, 1982). Further, women in England from the working class with children under 6 years of age were at greater risk of depression than women with children from the middle class (Brown & Harris, 1978).

## Conclusions

Depression is such a pervasive phenomenon that it has been called "the common cold of mental illness." Depression is likely to occur in approximately 25% of women in the United States at some point in their lives. Women experience depression twice as often as men, and twice as many women as men are hospitalized for depression.

By far the most frequent type of depression seen in mental health clinics is major depression; the second most common type is bipolar depression. There are a number of conditions associated with major depression, the most prominent of which is anxiety. Fortunately, with a structured interview one can elicit the critical differences between anxiety and depression, namely, fear of danger for anxious people and self-deprecating thoughts and negative attitudes for depressed people. In addition to anxiety, alcohol abuse is one of the most common clinical presenting problems associated with depression. Experts feel that treatment of the alcoholism is often the first clinical problem to attack, since the depressive symptomatology often abates if the drinking stops.

Many medications can cause depressive symptoms; two common causes are antihypertensives and steroids. The clinician should always be wary about this possibility. Physical conditions can also produce symptoms of depression; indeed, medical conditions contributing to depressive symptomatology are easily missed in clinical assessments.

Demographic risk factors associated with major depressive disorder are being female; being between the ages of 18 and 44, having been born after 1945; and being single, separated, widowed, or divorced.

Another clinical problem associated with depression is marital discord. Indeed, about half of depressed patients present with marital problems. Our own longitudinal research as well as that of others has indicated that marital problems are more likely to cause depression than depression is to cause marital problems. This point will be elaborated throughout this book, and we believe that treating the marital problems when depression and marital discord coexist is likely to be critical in producing an optimal outcome.

# 2

## Models of Depression

While many psychologists and psychiatrists have proffered what they described as theories of depression, most of these attempts would not meet the rigorous criteria for a theory. There are several general integrated accounts of depression (e.g., Akiskal, 1979; Lewinsohn, Hoberman, Terri, & Hautzinger, 1985) that attempt to encompass biological, psychological, and social variables; however, there have been no empirical tests of these integrated models *qua* models. More germane to our presentation, various psychologists and psychiatrists have presented what amount to unifactor models of depression. When one considers what is generally known about depression, the accounts are usually rather narrow, covering some particular psychological, biological, or sociological aspect of depression. Indeed, later we will also present our own account of marital discord and depression, and this account, also, is simply one model of depression. Even in cases in which marital discord is a key etiological factor, other variables, such as severe economic hardship or genetic predisposition to depression, may be relevant contributory etiological factors. Thus it is often useful to be aware of other unifactor models of depression and their likely relevance for a particular case of depression even when one is being guided primarily by the marital discord model. In addition, many of the unifactor models are associated with treatment recommendations that can be easily incorporated within a dyadic approach. Thus familiarity with the nonmarital models of depression will often suggest additional useful dyadic interventions to the clinician working with a depressed and discordant population.

Depression has been explained primarily by biological models and psychological models. The biological or biochemical models of depression predominated during the 1950s and 1960s, and individual psychological accounts of depression became accepted in the 1970s and 1980s. During the same time period, psychological and sociological models emphasizing stress, support, and coping became increasingly well developed. Finally, in the 1980s, another set of models of depression have received increasing attention, namely, the interpersonal models, especially the marital discord model of depression. While macrosocial and anthropological accounts have not had great impact in mental health circles to date, they appear to have a role in explaining depression. Accordingly, we will also briefly discuss explanations of depression that emanate from consideration of these larger-scale cultural and institutional factors. Given the diversity of influences on depression, as well as the variety of potential interventions that might be expected to have some impact on depression, a "models approach to psychotherapy" seems most appropriate for guiding therapy with depression (Beach, Abramson, & Levine, 1981).

## A Models Approach to Psychotherapy

A models approach to psychotherapy explicitly recognizes that a number of different unifactor models might have a role in accounting for a given syndrome of maladaptive behavior (Beach et al., 1981; Levine & Sandeen, 1985). Moreover, it is assumed that any given model provides a complete account for only some subgroup of individuals with a given syndrome. For depression, in particular, a models approach to psychotherapy seems appropriate. In the case of depression, several unifactor models in combination typically will be useful in accounting for the development and maintenance of a particular episode for a given individual. In turn, these models will be clinically useful when they are empirically verified and contain one or more elements that can be influenced through some form of clinical intervention. Each element highlighted by the model that can be influenced through clinical activity can be viewed as a possible point of therapeutic intervention. Because different models suggest different points of clinical intervention, the clinician's job is to decide how well a model fits for a particular patient and identify the most relevant set of intervention points for each client.

When more than one model seems necessary to capture the relevant contributory causes for a particular client or patient, it is important that the clinician be able to integrate points of intervention derived from other models into the overall treatment plan. From a clinical standpoint, it is not necessary to intervene at every available intervention point. However, intervention targeted at multiple intervention points may tend to enhance treatment outcome. The material that follows provides an overview of the main models of depression with empirical support. The marital discord model of depression is further explicated in Chapter 3. Thus it is our intent to provide the reader with an overview of the many unifactor models of depression that may be relevant for particular depressed persons and then to discuss in more detail the marital discord model of depression, which most directly informs our own approach to treatment.

## Biological Models of Depression

## Genetic Models

The results of family risk studies are among the most frequently cited reasons for viewing depression as resulting from biological factors. Based on research in the 1960s by Perris (1966) and Winokur, Clayton, and Reich (1969), it was generally concluded that affective disorders tend to be familial and that they should be subdivided into two types with apparently different patterns of familial transmission, namely bipolar and unipolar disorders (Rice et al., 1987). We will discuss both the family studies and the twin studies that have followed from this pioneering work.

### FAMILY STUDIES

The role of family or genetic factors was addressed long ago by Burton in *Anatomy of Melancholy* (1624/1973), in which he noted that the "inbred cause of melancholy is our temperature, in whole or part, which we receive from our parents" and "such as the temperature of the father is, such is the son's, and look what disease the father had when he begot him, his son will have after him?" (p. 184).

Over 350 years later, the role of family factors in depression was addressed in a major collaborative study in the United States (Andreasen et al., 1987). In what was called the National Institute of Mental Health Collaborative Study of the Psychobiology of Depression, a large number of standardized instruments were developed to assess prevalence and incidence of depression, life histories, psychosocial stressors, and outcome of depression. Of 955 subjects originally obtained from Boston, Chicago, Iowa City, New York, and St. Louis, 612 were entered into a family study; 3,423 of their first-degree relatives (children, siblings, and parents) were also assessed. The subjects, called probands, were divided into the following groups:

1. Schizoaffective: bipolar      $N = 37$
2. Schizoaffective: depressed      $N = 18$
3. Bipolar I (mania and depression)      $N = 151$
4. Bipolar II (hypomania and depression)      $N = 76$
5. Unipolar (major depressive disorder)      $N = 330$

Eighty percent of the subjects, or probands, were inpatients, while 20% were outpatients. Below, we will only discuss the family studies of unipolar and bipolar depressives.

Relatives of bipolar I probands had a higher rate of bipolar I illness (3.9%) than relatives of unipolar probands (0.6%). However, relatives of unipolar probands did not have a significantly higher rate of unipolar illness (28.4%) than relatives of bipolar (I and II) probands (24.5%). In an earlier study the average rate of unipolar depression among relatives of unipolar depressives was 16.6%, whereas the average rate of unipolar depression among relatives of bipolar (I and II) depressives was 15.6% (Gershon et al., 1982). Taken together, these studies indicate that there is a group of persons with largely bipolar family histories who are displaying symptoms that would lead to a diagnosis of unipolar depression for themselves. Conversely, persons with largely unipolar family histories do not appear to be at increased risk for bipolar depression. Thus the conclusions regarding the different patterns of familial transmission for bipolar and unipolar disorders have received increasing support over time.

In a large-scale adoption study in Denmark, Wender and colleagues (1986) were able to track index cases, or target cases, of individuals who had been hospitalized for unipolar depression. In addition, all the pertinent psychiatric and death records of each of the biological and adoptive parents were obtained for children adopted between 1924 and 1947. The likelihood that a relative of an index case (relative of a person with unipolar depression) would develop a depressive disorder was 2.1%, whereas the likelihood that a relative of a control subject would develop a depressive disorder was 0.3%. As Wender and colleagues (1986) noted, there was an eightfold increase in the likelihood of unipolar depression among biological relatives of depressed persons. Further, they found a fifteenfold increase in the likelihood of suicide in the relatives of depressed individuals. While this sample in Denmark had a much lower rate of depression in the control group than is seen in the United States, the authors pointed out that their method of ascertaining depression through records yields less depression than does the interview technique. Of course, it simultaneously yields a much more severely affected population than the full group of individuals with major affective disorder. Thus the large increase in risk of depression for the relatives of hospitalized patients with more severe depressive disorder in this investigation may be generalizable only to severely depressed patients and their biological relatives, not to the relatives of depressed patients with less severe depression. Nevertheless, the results clearly point to a tendency for severe depression to run in families and highlight the likely influence of a genetic predisposition or diathesis in these cases.

In summary, it should be clear that relatives of bipolar depressed persons and of those persons hospitalized with severe depression have an increased risk of developing depressive disorders. It appears that no matter whose research is used, first-degree relatives of bipolars have a much greater relative risk of developing bipolar depression than first-degree relatives of unipolar depressives have of developing unipolar depression. In addition, it appears that the genetic factors producing bipolar disorder will sometimes contribute to a disorder indistinguishable from the more common unipolar disorder. There is a two- to threefold increase in major depression in the first-degree relatives of more severely depressed persons, and the earlier the onset of the depression, the greater the prevalence of affective disorders in relatives (Weissman, 1987). However, it is unclear whether there is a significant increase in the risk of depression in the first-degree relatives of individuals suffering from mild to moderate depression. Thus, family studies suggest that a genetically transmitted diathesis for depression may be an important contributing factor for many cases of depression, particularly for persons with strong family histories of bipolar disorder or severe depression.

The family risk studies must be interpreted with caution, for they tend to overestimate the significance of genetic factors in influencing the rates of a disorder. It is possible that genetic factors account for the increased risk in first-degree relatives, but it is also possible that family factors of a nongenetic nature (e.g., modeling, poor parenting, lack of family structure, poor family problem solving) account for the increased risk in some cases. The family studies, however, provide an excellent lead to follow in studies of twins, where the influence of genetic factors can be assessed more directly. Even in twin studies, however, the role of genetic factors is probably not best studied in isolation. Given what is currently known, it seems likely that high-stress adoptive families would be much more likely to have high-risk children who subsequently develop disorders than low-stress adoptive families (cf. Tienari et al., 1985). Unfortunately, there has been little cross-fertilization to date between research on genetic factors in depression and on the role of family environment in depression.

## TWIN STUDIES

Twin studies of affective disorders have shown a statistically significant relationship between unipolar depression and genetic variables. Research with unipolar depressives yields monozygotic concordance rates of about 40% and dizygotic concordance rates of about 10% (Allen, 1976). A concordance rate refers to the likelihood of one twin's having a disorder given that the other twin has it. With bipolar disorders, the monozygotic concordance rates are about 70%, whereas the dizygotic concordance rates are only about 10% to 20% (Nurnberger & Gershon, 1982). Thus, given current population characteristics, one can better predict the occurrence of bipolar disorder from genotype than one can predict the occurrence of unipolar depression from genotype. This conclusion fits well with conclusions drawn from family studies. Accordingly, one would expect the genetic diathesis model to play a lesser role in accounts of unipolar depression than in accounts of bipolar depression.

Research with nonhospitalized twins from the general population in Australia has been used to help further unravel the contribution of genetic and environmental factors to general psychopathology, and to depression and anxiety in particular (Kendler, Heath, Martin, & Eaves, 1987). Genetic factors accounted for approximately 30% of the variance in both female and male depression, while environmental factors accounted for 36% of the variance in depression for both sexes. Of special interest in this research is the conclusion that the genetic factor is a nonspecific diathesis whereas the environmental factors are quite specific for symptoms of depression. Alternatively stated, these results suggest that the genetically transmitted diathesis for depression may be a nonspecific negative affectivity or reactivity to negative environmental events. This would imply that environmental events may be *more* rather than less consequential in producing fluctuations in level of depressive symptomatology for persons with a strong genetic diathesis for unipolar depression. Thus, even when a particular depressed individual appears to have a strong genetic diathesis for anxiety and/or depression, other unifactor models may nevertheless be relevant for a full understanding of the episode.

In brief, from both family studies and twin studies of depressed individuals and their relatives, it is clear that genetic factors play a role in the transmission of depression. However, while genetic factors appear to contribute significantly to depressive symptoms in nonhospitalized populations, environmental factors appear to account for equivalent amounts of depressive symptomatology. Thus, even for persons with an apparently strong genetic diathesis for depression, there is little reason to believe their depressions are inevitable or independent of their environment and how they perceive it.

A major drawback of the genetic model of depression is the failure of researchers to specify the inheritance characteristic that results in the increased vulnerability to depression. At present it seems plausible to assume that the inherited characteristic is a diathesis or risk for depression and/or anxiety that interacts with environmental stressors, such as marital and social stressors. This type of diathesis–stress model of depression may help focus the next generation of researchers on identifying the particular stressors most damaging to individuals with a genetic diathesis for depression.

## Biochemical Models

### NEUROENDOCRINE

In the last decade, there has been an explosion of research on the role of endocrine abnormality in depression. The bulk of the research has focused on a particular abnormality called dexamethasone nonsuppression. Some depressed patients produce an excess of cortisol and are unable to suppress this excessive cortisol secretion when given dexamethasone, a drug that suppresses cortisol secretion in most people (Arana, Baldessarini, & Ornsteen, 1985). This excess cortisol secretion and the inability to suppress cortisol when given dexamethasone is thought to relate to a defect in the pituitary, hypothalamus, or higher command centers governing these glands. Further, since messages sent from other parts of the brain to the hypothalamus use the norepinephrine system, it is also possible that during depressive episodes there is a more general dysfunction in norepinephrine transmission (Andreasen, 1984).

The knowledge about excess cortisol secretion among depressed persons has led to a series of studies about the potential value of using a diagnostic test to evaluate cortisol secretion in depressed persons. More specifically, it is now known that all humans have a circadian rhythm of cortisol secretion, with four to six major secretory episodes in a 24-hour period. The majority of these secretions occur in the morning for nondepressed individuals; after the morning burst of cortisol secretion, there is a gradual abatement of activity, with very little cortisol secretion late in the evening (Schlesser, 1986). On the other hand, some depressed people have 10 to 12 major cortisol secretory episodes, and the cumulative cortisol activity is higher than for nondepressed persons (Sachar, 1982). This knowledge about cortisol secretion and the information that dexamethasone will completely suppress cortisol secretion in almost all nondepressed persons but not in all depressed persons led to the development of the dexamethasone suppression test (DST; Carroll et al., 1981). One milligram of dexamethasone is given orally at 11 P.M., and cortisol levels are measured at 8 A.M., 4 P.M., and 11 P.M. on the following day. Nonsuppression is said to occur if at any of the three assessments, cortisol secretion exceeds a certain level.

Carroll and colleagues (1981) found that 67% of inpatients with endogenous depression (i.e., involving early morning awakening, loss of appetite and weight, and agitation or lethargy) had a positive DST, whereas only 4% of normal controls had a positive DST (i.e., their cortisol secretion was not suppressed with dexamethasone). The DST was thought to be of value in diagnosing depression and in predicting responsiveness to treatment. However, since other studies suggest that only 45% of depressed patients ever show dexamethasone nonsuppression (Arana et al., 1985) and only 25% show blunted thyrotropin response (Loosen, 1985), another widely studied endocrine abnormality, it may not always be necessary to invoke endocrine abnormality as part of one's account of a particular episode of depression for a given individual. Further, nonsuppression has not been found consistently to predict responsiveness to antidepressant medication for unipolar depressives, and there are no published studies showing that DST can predict the outcome of psychotherapy in unipolar depressives. However, persons showing DST abnormalities are unlikely to show a positive response to placebo, and some believe that an abnormal DST indicates the need for biological treatment (Joyce & Paykel, 1989). Others believe that while research continues on the clinical utility of the DST in conjunction with other biological measures, it should at present be thought of as primarily a research tool. Nevertheless, this line of research as well as a similar line of research on thyrotropin-releasing hormone (TRH) has indicated that a sizable group of depressed patients do show neuroendocrine abnormalities during their depressive episodes, and these abnormalities may mediate some aspects of their experience of depression. Thus this work can be viewed as supportive, in a general way, of the use of somatic interventions in this subset of depressions.

Interestingly, the DST may have a use as a means of monitoring success in treatment, since it tends to go to normal when the patient no longer feels depressed. Of course, this information also suggests that the

DST may be a state-dependent measure rather than a way to identify a characteristic that predisposes depressives to future episodes of depression.

## NEUROCHEMICAL

It is now believed that there are two types of depressions that result from chemical imbalances: norepinephrine-deficiency depressions and serotonin-deficiency depressions. Measurement of metabolites, or inactive products of neurotransmitters, has enabled researchers to study brain activities in intriguing ways. They can hypothesize that certain neurochemicals or neurotransmitters that aid in the transmission of electrical impulses in the brain have abnormalities. It is known that neurotransmitters operate in a fairly exact fashion: A specific amount of neurotransmitter is produced for aiding in the transmission of electrical impulses in the brain; the remainder that is not used is destroyed or rendered inactive. These latter cast off substances are called metabolites.

The main metabolite of norepinephrine is a chemical MHPG (3-methoxy-4-hydroxyphenylglycol), and the main metabolite of serotonin is 5-HIAA (5-hydroxyindoleacetic acid). Abnormalities of these metabolites have been found in the urine, blood, and spinal fluid of depressed persons. Urinary and blood assessments of metabolites have been found to be influenced by many factors that may render them inaccurate. Therefore spinal fluid analyses have become the method of choice in this research. However, data now seem to indicate that there are very strong correlations among measures of norepinephrine in the cerebrospinal fluid, plasma, and urine of persons who are cortisol nonsuppressors (Roy, Pickar, DeJong, Karoum, & Linnoila, 1988), suggesting that for this subpopulation of depressives one might be able to utilize urinary or blood measures effectively. Of potential relevance in treatment, it has been found that some antidepressants, such as desipramine, operate to enhance norepinephrine transmission and other medications, such as fluoxetine, enhance serotonin transmission. Thus, if depressions could be reliably subtyped according to the primary neurotransmitter anomaly, the choice of antidepressant theoretically would follow. However, research is conflicting on whether there is one group of depressed individuals who are low MHPG and normal 5-HIAA and another group of depressives who are low 5-HIAA and normal MHPG (Davis et al., 1988). Thus, while future developments in the study of neurotransmitter metabolites may have practical implications for the matching of particular pharmacotherapy interventions with particular types of depression, none are forthcoming at present. Nevertheless, the evidence does indicate that for many depressed patients substantial alteration in neurotransmitter activity occurs concurrently during their depression, and this altered activity may directly mediate many of the disturbing symptoms of depression.

## PHARMACOLOGICAL INTERVENTION

Pharmacological interventions for unipolar depression have sometimes been justified in popular publications on the basis of their purported role in normalizing a genetically determined biochemical defect or imbalance that often autonomously produces the depressive episode (Gold, 1987). Clearly, the evidence reviewed does not support this extreme biological characterization of unipolar depression. However, since neurotransmitters may directly mediate many of the behaviors affected in depression (e.g., sleep, appetite, pleasure) and since neurotransmitter level and activity are disturbed as a concomitant of many episodes of depression, the use of antidepressant agents that influence neurotransmitter level or activity should be helpful in reducing or eliminating symptoms of depression even if the disturbance in neurotransmitter level or activity is itself the result of environmental or cognitive changes. In addition, there is considerable direct evidence that antidepressants can be useful in the treatment of depression in many cases (Hollon & Beck, 1978; Klerman, 1988). In controlled trials, both the most recently developed as well as the older forms of antidepressants provide improvement rates of 66% to 75%, in contrast to placebos, which show improvement rates of 30% to 60%. However, exactly for whom they will work and exactly how or why they work is still not entirely clear (Baldessarini, 1988). Thus, while referral for medication will be appropriate for some depressed individuals, particularly for the more severely depressed, this should be viewed as a way of directly reducing a variety of depressive symptoms rather than addressing etiological factors of a psychological nature that may have produced the depressive episode. Likewise, it cannot be assumed that receiving antidepressant medication will provide any prophylaxis against subsequent episodes of depression once the medication is discontinued.

At present, antidepressant medication remains a very viable means of relieving depressive symptomatology in many cases; there is no reliable way, however, to match type of medication to type of depressed patient via biochemical assessment. The best-established predictors of positive response to antidepressant medication continue to include (1) an acute onset episode with melancholic features, (2) the depressed phase of a bipolar disorder, (3) prior successful treatment using antidepressant medication (Baldessarini, 1988)—all of which are best assessed via careful diagnostic interview.

## Psychological Models of Depression

### Cognitive Models

We will now review the major individual psychological conceptualizations of depression. Several of these theories are of a cognitive or a cognitive-behavioral nature and have considerable overlap with one another. In order to emphasize the central themes of the various cognitive theories of depression, these theories are reviewed under the headings that depict their central theme. Those themes, or central ingredients of the theories, are as follows:

- Cognitive distortions and negative self-schemata
- Negative attributions
- Reinforcement
- Script disruption and self-focus
- Self-control
- Problem solving and coping

#### COGNITIVE DISTORTIONS AND NEGATIVE SELF-SCHEMATA

According to Beck (1967, 1972, 1976), cognitive distortions cause many if not most of a person's depressed states. Three of the most important cognitive distortions are the following.

1. *Arbitrary inference.* Arbitrary inference refers to the process of drawing a conclusion from a situation, event, or experience when there is no evidence to support the conclusion or when the conclusion is contrary to the evidence. For example, an individual concludes that his boss hates him because he seldom says positive things to him.

2. *Overgeneralization.* Overgeneralization refers to an individual's pattern of drawing conclusions about his/her ability or performance or worth based on a single incident. An example of overgeneralization is that an individual concludes that she is worthless because she is unable to find her way to a particular address (even though she has numerous other exemplary skills).

3. *Magnification and minimization.* Magnification and minimization refer to errors in evaluation that are so gross as to constitute distortions. Most importantly, the magnifications refer to exaggeration

of negative events and minimization of positive events. Regarding magnification, for example, an individual who has a minor car accident erroneously concludes that the car is a total wreck and that a new car will have to be purchased. Regarding minimization, for example, an individual who receives positive feedback about his performance on a job minimizes the comment, saying that the person making the judgment had no idea how long he had to work to get the job done.

According to Beck, there are three important aspects of these distortions or depressive cognitions. First, they are automatic, that is, they occur without reflection or forethought. Second, they appear to be involuntary. Some patients indicate that these thoughts occur even though they resolved not to have them. Third, interestingly, the depressed person accepts these thoughts as plausible, even though others would clearly not view them in the same manner.

The general premise that depressed persons operate with a negative cognitive bias has been confirmed in a number of different contexts. That depressed persons have high levels of negative cognitions has been confirmed by the development and validation of the Automatic Thoughts Questionnaire (Hollon & Kendall, 1980). Depressed persons also endorse more depressogenic attitudes on scales such as Jones's Irrational Beliefs Test (Nelson, 1977) and the Dysfunctional Attitudes Scale (Weissman & Beck, 1978). There is also evidence that depressed persons endorse more self-deprecating statements and use more illogical justification for causal beliefs than do nondepressed persons (Cook & Peterson, 1986).

A second major premise of Beck's theory is that depressed persons have negative schemata regarding themselves. These schemata serve as means of processing and organizing information. Depression is said to occur as a result of activation of depressive schemata. The activation process of schemata held to originate in childhood is described as follows:

> During their development and maturation, people develop a large number of schemata that organize different aspects of experience. The schemata ostensibly undergo modification as a result of living, learning and experiencing. The formal characteristics of most depressogenic schemata, including the psychologically simplistic and "childish" content of the premises, the rigid directives, and their apparent lack of differentiation, all combine to create the impression that we are dealing with relatively stable, developmentally early constructions. . . . Most schemata contain erroneous conclusions which stem from the patient's earlier years and which have remained fairly constant through years of living. (Kovacs & Beck, 1978, p. 529)

Depression is hypothesized to occur when there is (1) vulnerability resulting from depressive schemata and (2) specific stresses, especially stresses that resemble earlier experiences that promoted the learning of depressive schemata, for example, the death of close relative in childhood. As Kovacs and Beck (1978) further pointed out, "The schema may be reactivated by conditions that the adult interprets as constituting irreversible loss such as the disruption of an interpersonal relationship" (p. 529).

While there is ample empirical support for the association of depression and negative cognitive factors, such as cognitive distortions, irrational beliefs, and negative statements about one's self, only now is there beginning to be research that demonstrates the ability of cognitive variables to predict subsequent depression. For example, longitudinal research by Lewinsohn, Hoberman, and Rosenbaum (1988) indicated that depression-related cognitions as measured by the Personal Beliefs Inventory were predictive of developing depressive symptoms 8 months later, even after controlling for initial levels of depression. Likewise, only recently has the schema specific–stress aspect of Beck's model been examined with supportive results (e.g., Hammen, Ellicott, Gitlin, & Jamison, 1989; Olinger, Kuiper, & Shaw, 1987; Robins & Block, 1988). Thus one of the most central aspects of Beck's theory still requires more research. Accordingly, at present it appears that a cognitive vulnerability plays a role in symptom formation for at least some individuals and in the maintenance of ongoing episodes of depression for many, if not all, depressed persons (O'Hara, Rehm, & Campbell, 1982; Dent & Teasdale, 1988). However, at present, cognitive vulnerability can be said to be predictive only of developing depressive symptomatology; it cannot yet be stated definitively that it predicts nosological depression (Barnett & Gotlib, 1988).

*Cognitive Therapy.* It has become clear that altering cognitions and behavior in a cognitive-behavioral format can work to relieve an ongoing episode of depression (Dobson, 1989) and can reduce the likelihood of relapse more than the use of psychopharmacology alone (e.g., Simons, Murphy, Levine, & Wetzel, 1986; Kovacs, Rush, Beck, & Hollon, 1981). Thus, cognitive processes are, at a minimum reasonable targets of intervention in the treatment of many depressed patients. In addition, cognitive therapy appears to work well at decreasing depressive symptomatology in the depressed spouse even in the context of ongoing marital discord (Beach & O'Leary, 1986; O'Leary & Beach, 1990). Thus, for many depressed patients, interventions targeted at altering dysfunctional, negative automatic thoughts are likely to be useful.

NEGATIVE ATTRIBUTIONS

The concept of learned helplessness originally derived from a process in which animals that received unavoidable shocks quickly looked depressed (i.e., they cowered, became motorically retarded, and failed to learn more adaptive responses; Seligman, 1975). In brief, the learned helplessness model of depression stated that depression is a consequence of exposure to noncontingent aversive events (Seligman, 1975). In turn, it was held that when individuals are exposed to uncontrollable situations, they are likely to develop the belief that outcomes are independent of their actions. Finally, it was postulated that these beliefs are then generalized to situations that are in fact controllable. The learned helplessness model was extended to diverse research with humans, and that research quickly led to cognitive reformulations of the learned helplessness model. Attributions about behavior and events were perceived as central etiological factors in the development of depression. The attributional reformulation of depression (Abramson, Seligman, & Teasdale, 1978), along with formulations by Weiner and Litman-Adizes (1980), held that an individual's causal attributions for his/her helplessness predicted lack of self-esteem and the severity of the depressive reaction. Further, it was postulated that depressed persons have an attributional style that is internal, stable, and global (Seligman, Abramson, Semmel, & von Baeyer, 1979). More specifically, it was held that depressed persons attribute the causes of negative events to their own internal failings or incompetence. It was also held that depressed persons saw these causes for negative events as being stable and global in their lives.

Although the specific content of maladaptive attributions has been a matter of some disagreement, it is indisputable that the attributional model has had a very wide-ranging impact in clinical psychology. Attributional models of depression and marital discord became the subject of considerable research (cf. Fincham, Bradbury, & Grych, 1990, on marital discord, and Hammen, 1985, on depression).

Support for the attributional model of depression was garnered from a number of areas. Depressed persons appear to attribute negative outcomes or failure experience to such internal characteristics as incompetence (e.g., DeMonbreun & Craighead, 1977; Kuiper, 1978). In experimental studies, differences have been found between depressed and nondepressed persons in terms of perceived control over outcomes. Meta-analysis of locus of control studies has shown that depressed individuals tend to perceive events as less controllable than nondepressed individuals; that is, they view events as being controlled by external rather than internal factors (Benassi, Sweeney, & Dufour, 1988). Also, while the literature has been portrayed as inconsistent in the past, it is now clear that when studies have sufficient power to detect the relevant relationships, depression and the tendency to attribute causes to stable and global causes are found to be associated (Robins, 1988).

If we turn our attention to the critical role of attributions in the *etiology* of depression, however, the picture is much less clear. Attributions are not very stable across time, and they do not typically generalize across situations (Hammen, 1985). Furthermore, there is no consistent evidence that attributions about negative events predict nosological depression. In at least half a dozen studies on the predictive role of negative attributions in depression, such attributions have failed to serve a unique predictive role over and above an individual's initial depression level. Recently, however, attribution researchers have refined their instruments to include more exact tests of the diathesis stress component of the theory. In particular, it has been noted that, like Beck's model, the attributional model posits that the cognitive diathesis will exert its effect on the development of symptoms only when *relevant* stress occurs. In one of the best tests of this aspect of the model to date, Metalsky, Halberstadt, and Abramson (1987) found that college students with a negative attributional style for achievement events showed more enduring dysphoria in response to receiving a low grade than students without a negative attributional style. In addition, it was found that particular attributions for the grade mediated the effect of attributional style on enduring dysphoria. While this study and others now appearing in the literature do not establish the role of negative attributional style in predicting clinical or nosological depression, they point, at a minimum, to a role for attributional style in accounting for the development of depressive symptomatology. In addition, they suggest that future work utilizing similar strategies may uncover a role for attributional style in predicting nosological depression.

One possible problem with attributional explanations as they have been developed to date is that formulations regarding attributional styles have been derived from Weiner's theory of achievement motivation, and most of the research regarding consistency of attributional styles has taken place in achievement contexts. As Hammen (1985) has argued, however, some people may have issues that are more important to them than achievement. For example, some may be much more concerned about interpersonal loss. Along these lines, Barthe and Hammen (1981) did not find that depressed persons who had difficulty dealing with problems in romantic relationships had negative attributions that were stable and internal. For interpersonal relationships, other types of attributional processes, such as the attribution of blame, may be more important (Fincham, Beach, & Nelson, 1987). These findings may lead attributional researchers to again reformulate their models of negative cognition to include dimensions of attributional style that are much less integrally related to achievement contexts.

## REINFORCEMENT

A script disruption model of depression has been advanced recently by Lewinsohn and colleagues (1985). We shall discuss this "cognitive" reformulation of the reinforcement model below. However, the earlier "behavioral" model (Lewinsohn & Arconad, 1981) has both simplicity and clarity to recommend it, and we include it here for its heuristic value. Lewinsohn's earlier behavioral model of depression had a primary focus on elevated rates of aversive events and a paucity of reinforcement. More specifically, the reinforcement model had three foci: (1) *availability* of few positive reinforcers and a surplus of punishers, (2) *skill deficiencies* that make it difficult for an individual to obtain positive reinforcers or to cope with negative events, and (3) *individual susceptibility* to negative events and a reduced impact of positive events.

In fact, Lewinsohn has provided reasonable support indicating that depressives do have more aversive events and less reinforcement than nondepressed persons. Further, this reinforcement model of depression has led to group treatments of depression that have repeatedly been found successful (Brown & Lewinsohn, 1984; Lewinsohn & Arconad, 1981; Lewinsohn, Antonuccio, Steinmetz, & Teri, 1984). Concern for the limitations of the original model, which emphasized overt positive and negative events, led to a new model, which posited a central role for disruption of scripted or automatic behavior patterns, leading to a focus on oneself and increased self-criticism. Nevertheless, the points of intervention highlighted by the original model are not contradicted by the new model and will often provide useful guidance to the clinician working with a depressed population.

## SCRIPT DISRUPTION AND SELF-FOCUS

The reformulation or extension of the earlier reinforcement model of depression has two clear assets, according to Hoberman and Lewinsohn (1985): (1) It takes into account the knowledge gleaned from treatment outcome research, and (2) it provides direction to practitioners interested in the development of maximally efficacious treatment programs. The model is an integrative one in that it is multifaceted and, as such, includes many aspects of a person and his/her environment that may predict depression. In addition, it has gone beyond the earlier reinforcement models to include cognitive factors and scripted behavior.

Scripted behavior has been discussed by psychologists and sociologists for many years. Scripts refer to well-learned patterns of social behavior. It is held by Lewinsohn and colleagues (1985) that when depression-evoking events occur, they disrupt these expected, automatic patterns of behavior and elicit an immediate negative emotional response (dysphoria). In turn, the emotional upset leads to behavioral changes, producing a reduced rate of positive reinforcement and/or elevated rate of aversive experience. If an individual is unable to reverse the depressogenic process, a heightened state of self-awareness is prompted that leads to self-criticism and withdrawal. The elicitation of the state of self-awareness is held to impede the ability to use protective self-enhancing cognitive schemata. This leaves the individual in a vicious cycle of depressogenic processes, a cycle in which attention to the self produces depression and depression leads to more self-focus.

Self-focus has become the subject of much research and discussion in the study of depression. Duval and Wicklund (1972) and Wicklund (1975) postulated that focusing attention on the self initiates a self-evaluative process by which one's present standing on a self-relevant dimension is compared with one's aspiration for that dimension. If one falls short of the standard, the self-focus produces negative affect. The self-focus literature was reviewed by Pyszczynski and Greenberg (1987), who presented both correlational and experimental evidence in support of the self-focusing style as a key factor in the maintenance or etiology of depression. The research on sex differences in depression has also been reviewed, and elevated self-focusing in females has been held to be a possible factor in the 2:1 ratio of depression for females and males (Nolen-Hoeksema, 1987).

Ingram and colleagues have found that elevated self-focusing levels characterize mild depression in both college samples and clinically depressed persons (cf. Ingram, Lumrey, Cruet, & Sieber, 1987). As Pyszczynski and Greenberg (1987) noted, the persistence in self-focusing occurs when there is a loss in the personal, social, or work sphere and when the loss is irreplaceable or of central importance to an individual. They proposed that "depression occurs to the extent that the individual who experiences a loss fails to disengage and continues to self-focus in the absence of any way to gain what was lost" (p. 127). In brief, self-focus concerning the loss persists long after the point at which it would have been adaptive to direct one's attention elsewhere. Given the available data, it seems reasonable to expect that when script disruption or other factors prompt increased self-focus for the depressed individual, there will be an intensification of dysphoria. In addition, it is reasonable to expect that clinical interventions that draw attention away from a self-focus should tend to rather rapidly elevate mood. It is to be hoped that more direct clinical tests of interventions derived from this model will be forthcoming.


## SELF-CONTROL

A general self-control model of behavior has been presented by Kanfer (1970) and adapted to depression by Rehm (1977, 1987). Basically, the positions of Kanfer and Rehm are that when an individual notices that

> some form of behavior is not functioning well or will not be able to achieve desired outcomes, a self-monitoring, self-evaluation, self-reinforcement feedback sequence is engaged. Self-monitoring involves observation of one's own performance including its antecedents, consequences, and concomitants. Information regarding one's performance is then compared to an external standard. (Rehm, 1987, p. 10)

In addition, it is held that a self-attribution process is set in motion in which an individual judges his/her positive behavior as worthy of praise if the behavior is internally caused. Similarly, negative behavior is judged as blameworthy if internally caused.

In Rehm's view, the triad of deficits that are central to the development of depression are those involved in self-monitoring, self-evaluation, and self-reinforcement. Let us evaluate the evidence for the role of each of these concepts in the maintenance and etiology of depression.

*Self-Monitoring.* According to Rehm (1977), depressed persons selectively attend to negative outcomes and to immediate rather than delayed outcomes. As discussed earlier in this chapter in several contexts, there is evidence to support the view that depressed persons attend more to negative events than to positive events. On the basis of a series of studies (DeMonbreun & Craighead, 1977), it appears that the most consistent finding in this literature is underestimation of positive feedback, especially when given at high rates.

On the other hand, evidence is equivocal regarding attention to immediate rather than delayed outcomes (Rehm & Plakosh, 1975). Of special interest as a challenge to the etiological role of selectively attending to negative events was a study by O'Hara and Rehm (1979) in which they asked subjects to specifically attend to and record positive or negative events over the course of a 4-week period. To the investigators' surprise, the change in the subjects' moods that had been predicted by their recording of positive and negative events did not occur (O'Hara & Rehm, 1979).

*Self-Evaluation.* According to Rehm (1977), depressed persons set standards for themselves that are excessively stringent. They are too pessimistic. The standard may be too high in an absolute sense or too high relative to their own skills and abilities. There are many clinical anecdotes about depressed individuals' having standards that are too high, but the evidence for the comparatively high standards is relatively meager. In one study, depressed persons rated their performances as poor even though their performances were identical to those of nondepressed persons (Loeb, Beck, & Diggory, 1971). In a related study, there was an association between the setting of high standards and low self-esteem in males (Warren, 1976). While these studies indirectly provide supportive evidence for the causative role of excessively high standards in the etiology of depression, there has simply not been enough direct testing of this hypothesis to allow one to place strong credence in it.

*Self-Reinforcement.* Self-reinforcement occurs less frequently in depressed college students than in nondepressed students (Nelson & Craighead, 1977), and depressed psychiatric patients reinforce themselves less on memory tasks than do nondepressed subjects. Further, depressed patients also punish themselves more than do nondepressed subjects. In brief, self-reinforcement does appear to operate differently for depressed than for nondepressed persons.

Rehm's self-control model of depression has led to a series of therapy outcome studies of depression in which depressives have been successfully treated (O'Leary & Wilson, 1987). Taken together, the data suggest that self-monitoring, self-evaluation, and self-reinforcement are problematic in depression. In addition, it appears that changing all these parameters together can influence depression. However, it remains unclear that these variables play an etiological role in nosological depression.

## PROBLEM SOLVING AND COPING

A number of authors have recently suggested that depression may be understood as a failure to cope with ongoing life problems or stressors. It has been hypothesized that coping effectively with problems and stressors can moderate the impact of these problems and help prevent them from becoming chronic (Billings & Moos, 1982). In addition, it appears that coping mediates the emotional response produced by a variety of psychosocial stressors (Folkman & Lazarus, 1988). Generally, research has divided coping strategies into those which are problem focused and those which are emotion focused. Problem-focused coping is indicated for those situations that are appraised as changeable, while emotion-focused coping is indicated when a problem situation is appraised as unchangeable (Lazarus & Folkman, 1986). A third category of coping strategy has been called perception-focused coping (Pearlin & Schooler, 1978). This category would include those cognitive strategies designed to alter the meaning of a situation to reduce its perceived threat value. Let us evaluate the evidence for the problem-solving and coping model of depression.

Depressed patients show a lower likelihood of rapid recovery if they display poor coping skills (Parker, Brown, & Blignault, 1986). Avoidance coping strategies appear to be particularly likely in depression and predict nonremission of depression (Krantz & Moos, 1988). Depressed persons also show elevated levels of emotion-focused coping strategies, such as wishful thinking, distancing, self-blame, and isolation, relative to community controls (Kuiper & Olinger, 1989). It has also been reported that depressed individuals show both more hostile confrontive coping and more self-control coping aimed at holding hostile feelings in check, as well as elevated levels of avoidance (Folkman & Lazarus, 1986). This suggests a tendency for depressed persons to use conflicting or self-defeating coping strategies. Interestingly, only self-isolation, an interpersonal avoidance strategy, appears to be an enduring coping style of persons vulnerable to depression (Kuiper & Olinger, 1989). Thus coping processes appear to change for the worse during an episode of depression, and poor coping helps to maintain the episode. In particular, depressed persons appear likely to avoid problem situations and to engage in strategies with a low likelihood of resulting in problem resolution or an enhanced sense of personal control.

A social problem-solving model of depression has been proposed which attempts to integrate much of the coping and cognitive literatures on depression (Nezu, Nezu, & Perri, 1989). The problem-solving model highlights the following components of successful problem-solving coping:

1. Problem orientation. A good problem-solving orientation includes the ability to recognize problems, to accept problems as normal, to engage problems constructively rather than avoid them or engage in maladaptive habitual behaviors, and to expect that problem solving can be successful.
2. Problem definition. Optimal problem definition involves seeking relevant information, describing information clearly, differentiating

facts from assumptions, identifying the key elements that make the situation problematic, and setting realistic problem-solving goals.
3. Generation of alternatives. This component of problem solving emphasizes brainstorming and deferral of judgment regarding particular suggested solutions.
4. Decision making. The goal of this component is to evaluate the possibilities generated and select the alternative that most nearly matches the problem-solving goals.
5. Solution implementation and verification. This component acknowledges the need for later evaluation of an implemented problem-solving strategy, highlighting the fact that problem solving is open-ended.

Recent research suggests that problem-solving styles are problematic in depression (e.g., Gotlib & Asarnow, 1979; Nezu, Nezu, Saraydarian, Kalmar, & Ronan, 1986; Nezu & Ronan, 1987). In addition, a problem-solving therapy approach appears promising as a treatment modality for depression (Nezu & Perri, 1989). Thus remediation of coping and problem-solving styles should be considered potentially useful clinical approaches in the treatment of depression. When successful, therapy aimed at enhancing coping and problem solving should decrease the length of a depressive episode. Additional work is necessary, however, both to disclose an etiological role for coping and problem-solving deficits in depression and to demonstrate the ability of enhanced coping and problem-solving skills in protecting against subsequent episodes of depression.

## Interpersonal Models

The major focus of this book will be interpersonal factors in depression, especially marital factors. Accordingly, Chapter 3 contains a review of additional material on social support and interpersonal factors in depression as they relate to marital discord. However, in order to provide a comprehensive overview of factors that contribute to depression, several interpersonal models and their role in depression will be covered here briefly. These models are as follows: (1) anger turned inward, (2) social support, (3) marital discord, (4) coercion, and (5) family systems.

### ANGER TURNED INWARD

Psychoanalytic views of depression have typically emphasized loss of love and emotional security as a key variable in depression (Klein, 1940), as postulated in Freud's (1917/1986) classic paper "Mourning and Melancholia." Since the original presentation by Freud, however, psychodynamic theorists have placed more weight on loss of self-esteem than on loss of another or loss of another's love (Arieti & Bemporad, 1978). The essence of Freud's view was that a loss produces self-criticism and castigation and that, in turn, the individual becomes angry with him/herself. This process was said to occur because the individual becomes angry at the lost person, but because hostility or anger toward the lost person would produce guilt, the individual directs the anger toward him/herself. The individual is held to be largely unaware of his/her hatred toward the lost object, and this hatred or anger is held to remain outside consciousness.

Partial evidence for the psychodynamic view of depression has been proffered from research on manifest dream content of depressives in which loss and failure are dominant themes. Interestingly, however, anger and hostility are not common dream themes (e.g., Beck & Hurvich, 1959). Another line of research into possible unconscious mechanisms in depression was the analysis of the content of free-association fantasies during psychoanalysis. Like the work on dream content, there was no evidence to support the notion that hostility was a critical issue. Instead, the most common themes were personal incompetence and failure (Beck, 1963). Beck's conclusion was that belief in incompetence, not internalized anger, was the most salient theme in the depressed person's distress (Hollon & Beck, 1979). Thus a major component of the original psychodynamic hypothesis was not confirmed.

Other partial support for the psychodynamic view of anger and depression is the research indicating that depressives often display intense overt anger with family members (Weissman, Klerman, & Paykel, 1971). Recent analyses by behavioral researchers of conditional probabilities of depressed and nondepressed persons also provide some support for the notion that depressed individuals display overt anger with their spouses (Biglan et al., 1985; Beach & Nelson, 1989a). Both found that depressed, discordant wives were more negative toward their spouses than were nondepressed, nondiscordant wives. However, the anger observed in these studies was overt rather than retroflected anger. Further, studies of depressives do not typically find that anger and depression are inversely related.

While the psychodynamic view of depression has been seriously questioned (cf. Hollon & Beck, 1979), it has prompted interesting research on melancholia, bereavement, anger, and depression. In addition, the interpersonal treatment (IPT) research of Klerman and Weissman clearly was influenced by neo-Freudians such as Fromm-Reichmann, Fromm, and Horney (Klerman, Weissman, Rounsaville, & Chevron, 1984).

*Interpersonal Psychotherapy.* This successful treatment approach emphasizes abnormal grief, interpersonal disputes, role transitions, loss, and interpersonal deficits, as well as social and familial factors. Recent results of a large, multicenter collaborative study conducted by NIMH have indicated that IPT can work as well as antidepressant medication for many depressed patients (Elkin et al., 1989). In addition, earlier research has indicated that IPT can improve the social functioning of depressed patients in a manner not typically produced by antidepressant medications alone (Weissman, Klerman, Paykel, Prusoff, & Hanson, 1974; DiMascio et al., 1979). As will be discussed below, these improvements in social functioning and interpersonal environment appear to be particularly important for depressed persons.

## SOCIAL SUPPORT

In sociological and social-psychological research, social support has taken on a wide variety of meanings. However, social support generally refers either to concrete aspects of social networks, such as size, density, and intensity, or else to the provisions offered by social contacts, such as expressive and instrumental support (Lin, 1986). Further, the positiveness or negativity of an individual's contacts with members of the social network is also considered a very important characteristic of the social network.

Research on whom individuals choose to confide in reveals that both females and males would most often turn to their spouses (Denoff, 1982). However, both males and females are more likely to turn to a female friend than a male friend (Lin, Woelfel, & Dumin, 1986). Depressed persons are less likely than nondepressed persons to have a large or dense friendship network, and there now is startling evidence that lack of social support is as strong a factor in predicting death as was smoking several years ago (House, Landis, & Umberson, 1988). There is considerable evidence of relationships among various aspects of social support and depression (Barnett & Gotlib, 1988). Despite these associations, the mechanism underlying these relationships is not always clear; general behavioral or affective abnormalities may impede the development of close interpersonal relationships (Kessler, Price, & Wortmann, 1985), or perhaps the relationship between social support and depression results from the fact that depressed persons do not seek social support (Kuiper & Olinger, 1989). Another interpretation is that depressed persons have an aversive interpersonal style that prompts others to reject or dislike them (Gotlib & Colby, 1987). These views regarding the lack of an affiliative tendency and aversive interpersonal style need not be conflicting. Indeed, they all can be partly true. Importantly, however, it appears that social network size and density may not be the most powerful aspect of social support; rather, it appears that the provisions of close relationships, such as emotional support and perceived availability of support, may be more powerful in buffering the effect of stress (Lin, Dean, & Ensel, 1986; Kessler & McLeod, 1985).

In the area of depression, several studies indicate the relevance of social support. The effects of general social support and strong ties with an intimate confidant were examined by Lin, Dean, and Ensel (1986). Using a longitudinal design, the authors assessed the independent roles of social support via relationships in general (weak tie support) and via close relationships (strong tie support) on the formation of depressive symptomatology. Social support was found to have a strong direct and independent effect on depression and its change across time. It was also found that social support buffered the effect of stress on symptom formation. Of particular interest, it was found that a close relationship with a confidant (typically a spouse) who was providing instrumental and expressive support was the strongest indicator of social support and the best predictor of subsequent depressive symptomatology.

In a previous study, Lin and Ensel (1984) assessed social support by asking respondents whether they had a close companion and enough close friends; again, the presence or absence of such social support showed a direct effect on change in level of depressive symptomatology. In a more specific domain, Cutrona (1984) assessed the level of social support available to women during their pregnancies. He found that level of general social integration as well as total support available predicted level of symptoms at 8 weeks postpartum, even after controlling for initial level of symptoms. Further indication of a relationship between depressive symptomatology and social support is provided by the finding that within an already depressed sample, lack of social support is a strong predictor of the strength of suicidal intent (Thomssen & Möller, 1988). Likewise, level of social adjustment following treatment (both pharmacotherapy and cognitive therapy) for depression has been found to be associated with relapse (Simons et al., 1986).

Thus there is a considerable amount of good prospective evidence linking lack of social support with the formation or maintenance of depressive symptomatology and suggesting a role of social support in buffering life stress. While there is some evidence that general social integration and certain structural features of the social network per se are helpful in maintaining positive mental health, stronger evidence links the absence of the provisions of close relationships with the development of depressive symptomatology. Accordingly, the work on general social support and depression can be seen as pointing in the direction of direct consideration of intimate relationships and their role in depression. Since the strongest family ties are usually in dyads such as the marital relationship, it is natural to look to the marital relationship for particularly powerful opportunities to provide social support (Burgess, 1981; Weiss, 1974).

## MARITAL DISCORD

There is considerable support for an association between marital discord and depression (Beach, Arias, & O'Leary, 1987; Coleman & Miller, 1975; Renne, 1970; Weiss & Aved, 1978). It had been expected by some that the association between marital discord and depression would be greater for women than men. However, the association between marital discord and depression is generally equivalent between sexes when one looks across studies. Indeed, Weissman (1987; see Table 2-1) reports that in a representative sample drawn from the New Haven area, the risk of having a major depressive episode was approximately 25 times higher for both males and females if they were in a discordant marital relationship than if they were in a nondiscordant marital relationship.

Another way to conceptualize the association between marital discord and depression is to look at this association in clinic samples. There appears to be about a 50% overlap of the association between marital discord and depression in samples selected for marital problems or in samples selected for depression (Beach et al., 1985; Rounsaville et al., 1979a, 1979b). While the amount of overlap between depression and marital problems may seem huge given the likelihood of the two problems occurring on the basis of chance alone, it has been known for almost 30 years that marital problems are among the most frequent problems for which adults seek treatment in a mental health facility. In 1960 Gurin, Veroff, and Feld found that 42% of individuals seeking treatment viewed their problems as marital. Similarly, in 1968 Sager, Gundlach, and Kremer found that approximately half of all patients who sought psychotherapy treatment did so because of marital problems. Thus the findings that marital problems have a significant impact on mood and the presence of a depressive disorder and that they figure prominently in the complaints of many depressed persons should not be surprising.

Retrospective research has helped illuminate the temporal relationship between depression and marital discord. For example, negative marital events often precede the onset of depressive symptoms (Paykel, 1979). In order to determine the ordering of marital discord and depression, Paykel and colleagues (1969) and Paykel and Tanner (1976) used semistructured interviews of hospitalized patients to determine event

TABLE 2-1. Six-Month Prevalence (Rates/100) of Major Depression

|  | Male | Female |
|---|---|---|
| Separated/divorced | 4.4% | 6.3% |
| Single | 2.4% | 3.9% |
| Married: Gets along with spouse | 0.6% | 2.9% |
| Married: Doesn't get along with spouse | 14.9% | 45.5% |
|  | Odds ratio[a] | |
| Odds of major depression for those who say they don't get along with spouse | 25.8 | 28.1 |

Note. From Weissman, M. M. (1987). Advances in psychiatric epidemiology: Rates and risks for major depression. *American Journal of Public Health*, 77, 448. Copyright 1987 by the American Public Health Association. Reprinted by permission of the publisher and author.
[a]Adjusted for age.

occurrence and event timing. In both cases, marital arguments and other stressors preceded depression and were especially prominent during the month preceding depression onset. Using a different methodology, Ilfeld (1976) had community couples make a judgment about the length of their depression, social stressors, and marital problems. Having the subjects judge the duration of various social stressors was done to minimize recall biases. On the average, marital distress was of considerably longer duration than the depressive symptomatology. These data in the aggregate support the proposition that marital problems are more likely to precede depression than vice versa. Using a retrospective interview approach, Brown and Harris (1978), studying working-class women in England, found that lack of a confiding relationship with a boyfriend or spouse was a significant vulnerability factor in the development of depression. Of special interest, they found that disturbed ties with a husband were related to a risk for depression only in the presence of other stressors. However, since some of their stressors were essentially marital stressors (e.g., husband's drinking), the Brown and Harris work may underestimate of the role of marital discord in the etiology of depression.

There is now also some prospective work examining the impact of marital variables on the development of depression. Monroe, Bromet, Connell, and Steiner (1986) found that with nonsymptomatic women in nondiscordant marriages, social support within a marriage predicts lower risk for depressive symptoms 1 year later. The role of marital discord on later increases in depressive symptoms has also been evident in our own longitudinal research (Beach, Arias, & O'Leary, 1988). With newly married couples, marital discord at 6 months predicted higher levels of depressive symptoms at 18 months, even after controlling for initial symptoms and intervening levels of life stress. Similarly, recent work by Markman and colleagues (Markman, Duncan, Storaasli, & Howes, 1987) indicates that women reporting marital problems very early in their relationship are at elevated risk for later depressive symptomatology.

Taken together the data lead one to the conclusion that marital problems play an important role in the etiology of depression. The retrospective and cross-sectional research would appear to link marital discord to *nosological* depression, while the longitudinal research to date demonstrates only that marital variables can predict future levels of depressive symptoms. Finally, recent evidence also links the presence of marital discord and perceived criticism by the spouse with relapse following successful somatic treatment for depression (Hooley & Teasdale, 1989). Thus marital discord emerges as a candidate for true etiological significance in depression on a par with any other variable studied to date. In Chapter 3 we return to the marital discord model of depression to provide additional elaboration.

## COERCION

The concept of coercion in psychology was developed by Patterson and Reid (1970), who noted that certain children's behavior, such as whining and temper tantrums, can be coercive in that they prompt parents to stop them by placating the child. Consequently, the child is reinforced for tantrums and the parent is reinforced for "giving in." This coercion model has been generalized to cover many family interactions, including marital interactions. In marriages, a depressed woman may often engage in aversive behavior, such as complaining about her life, and the husband may console her or stop making critical comments to her. This aversive behavior on the part of depressed individuals has been thought to be functional in reducing others' attacks and in obtaining positive social consequences (Biglan, Hops, & Sherman, 1988). In fact, Biglan and colleagues (1985) provided initial data supporting this functional role of depressive behavior. Similarly, Nelson and Beach (in press) found only a nonsignificant effect of aversive/depressive behavior on reducing critical comments of husbands in their depressed, maritally discordant sample, but a significant effect in their *nondepressed*, maritally discordant sample. Clearly, depressive behavior is related in some manner to the reduction of spousal aggression, and this represents a plausible reinforcer of depressive behavior. However, as Biglan and colleagues (1988) pointed out, considerable work is required before it can be asserted confidently

that the social consequences of depressive behavior are typically reinforcing and help maintain a depressed person's depressive behavior.

We do not view depressive behavior in general as simply a function
of operant contingencies in a dyadic relationship. It is possible, however,
that in certain situations an angry yet concerned husband may become
much less critical of his wife if she complains about her depressive
symptomatology. To the extent that this contingency increases her depressive behavior over time, the depressive behavior would be said to
have been straightforwardly reinforced. Since the coercive power of
depressive behavior to suppress critical comments by the spouse is negatively correlated with the duration of the marital discord (Nelson &
Beach, in press), it is possible that a discordant spouse may become
increasingly depressed as higher levels of depressive behavior are required
to continue to suppress his/her partner's critical behavior. This would
provide one mechanism linking longer marital discord with an increasing
probability of depression. In addition, it has been shown that significant
others can exert a direct effect on depressive behaviors via straightforward reinforcement and extinction procedures (Brannon & Nelson,
1987).

While the coercion model has not yet generated unequivocal support, neither has it been adequately tested. It also provides a powerful
framework for intervention if empirically confirmed. Accordingly, it is to
be hoped that additional work will be stimulated by the coercion model.


## FAMILY SYSTEMS

Systems views of depression have been presented by a number of individuals, but Coyne (1976) has articulated one of the most frequently cited
presentations of the systemic view of depression. Similar to the coercive
model presented above, Coyne maintains that the depressed person's
behavior is maintained or increased in part by his/her social environment. It is suggested that the depressed person demands attention
through complaints about the depression. A sympathetic spouse may
initially react with concern about the depressed person's feelings. However, according to Gotlib and Colby (1987):

> If the depressed person's symptomatic behavior continues, . . . others with
> whom they interact themselves begin to feel depressed, anxious, and frus-
> trated or hostile, feelings that are communicated subtly (and mixed with
> qualifiers) to the depressed person. When the depressed individual observes
> these negative or discrepant messages, she or he becomes increasingly symp-
> tomatic in an attempt to regain the initial support. (p. 17)

It is hypothesized that as this process continues, the depressed person "turns off" others, and he/she is eventually seen as a whiner or a complainer. In the extreme, these depressed individuals are simply avoided by others.

A good deal of data has been generated in an attempt to support Coyne's (1976) basic assertions. Using primarily stranger dyads, considerable evidence has been found that depressed patients prompt rejection, devaluation, and some sort of negative mood in the target of the interaction (e.g., Biglan, Rothlind, Hops, & Sherman, 1989). In addition, it is clear that spouses of depressed patients are themselves more depressed than persons in the general community (Coyne et al., 1987). However, it is not clear that this effect is specific to depression (Boswell & Murray, 1981). Further, the mediating mechanism of the rejection and devaluation of the depressed person by the nondepressed person does not seem to be induction of negative mood in the nondepressed person, as originally proposed by Coyne (cf. Gurtman, 1986). Instead, it seems that perceived dissimilarity of the depressed person to the nondepressed person may account for the rejection of and negative reactions to the depressed person (Rosenblatt & Greenberg, 1988). Interestingly, depressed individuals do not reject or devalue other depressed persons as much as nondepressed individuals reject depressed individuals (Rosenblatt & Greenblatt, 1988). Thus, if a husband and a wife are both depressed, they might not reject each other as much as would be the case if one member of the dyad were depressed and the other were not.

Considerable additional work is necessary to demonstrate the etiological significance of the processes highlighted in Coyne's model. In particular, longitudinal work with intimate dyads would seem necessary to capture the most important relationships being hypothesized. At present, no clear statement can be made regarding the role of such variables as indirect or ambiguous spousal negativity on the development or exacerbation of depressive symptomatology and nosological depression.

Couple-based intervention for depression has been proposed by systemically oriented theorists (e.g., Coyne, 1988, 1989). Similar to our own therapeutic approach, Coyne suggested a structured, goal-oriented, relatively brief intervention that includes homework, an awareness of depression-related symptoms, and attention to depression-related processes that can complicate marital therapy. Also similar to our approach, Coyne emphasized the importance of improved communication and intimacy in the marital dyad. Contrary to our approach, Coyne recommended the use of paradox, symptom prescription, and considerable use of split sessions in which the therapist meets with each spouse individually followed by a brief joint meeting. Unfortunately, empirical work on the utility of paradox and symptom prescription for couples with a depressed member is not currently available. Reframing, another technique suggested by Coyne, would appear to have some similarity to the reattribution techniques we discuss later. Reframing that emphasizes "positive" elements of problem behaviors may be a valuable technique in working with a variety of problems (Shoham-Salomon & Rosenthal, 1987).

## NEGATIVE LIFE EVENTS

It has been known for some time that significant life events are correlated with or associated with the onset of depression (Paykel, 1982). Since the Holmes and Rahe (1967) study, positive life events, such as marriage and job promotion, and negative life events, such as marital separation and failure to obtain a mortgage, have been studied in the context of stress research paradigms. In general, negative life events have accounted for most of the variance in depression and other psychopathology, with little to no variance accounted for by positive events. While the authors have occasionally seen depression following a promotion, such instances are truly rare, and comparison group research usually does not confirm the view of depression as caused by positive life events. Indeed, a contextual approach, such as that utilized by Brown and Harris (1978), will typically show that when "positive" events do appear to have precipitated a depressive episode, it is because when considered in context they can be seen as holding considerable threat for the individual. In accord with the material presented earlier on marital discord, in exactly half of the 12 studies summarized by Paykel (1982) marital separations were found to be related to depression. This finding is quite impressive, since separations are unlikely to occur at any given point in time.

Other negative events, such as bereavement and job loss, have also been associated with increased depressive symptomatology. In addition, early loss of a parent has been associated with later depressive symptomatology. Loss of a parent is not uniquely associated with depression, however; such loss is associated with generally elevated psychopathology. In addition, the relationship of loss of a parent and later depression appears to be mediated through its impact on loss of maternal care for the child (Brown, Harris, & Bifulco, 1986). In Paykel and colleagues' (1969) research, the following life events significantly differentiated depressed patients (100 outpatients, 30 day patients, 25 emergency unit patients, and 65 inpatients) and controls:

- Increase in arguments with spouse
- Marital separation
- Start of new type of work

- Change in work conditions
- Serious personal illness
- Death of immediate family member
- Serious illness of family member
- A family member's leaving home

"Increases in arguments with spouse," "marital separation," and "start of a new type of work" were the items most clearly differentiating the two groups.

The daily hassles that we encounter each day may also have a very significant impact on us. Noise, rush-hour traffic, minor arguments, or critical comments by a partner about relatively unimportant things may lead us to be depressed. In fact, in a middle-aged community sample, daily hassles were better predictors of depression than were major life events (Kanner, Coyne, & Schaefer, 1981). In a number of areas stress per se is not sufficient to produce psychopathology such as depression, alcohol abuse, or spouse abuse. Indeed, there are many individuals who can withstand extreme amounts of daily or major stress and not become depressed. This observation has led researchers such as Billings and Moos (1982) to view stress as a precipitating factor for depression operating within a larger theoretical context that includes personal resources (e.g., social skills and problem-solving ability) and environmental resources (e.g., material, emotional, and informational support from family and friends).

Thus there is considerable evidence linking stress to the onset of depression. While much has been made of the relatively low correlation between measures of stress and depression, Brown and Harris (1986) pointed out that this is exactly analogous to the relationship between cigarette smoking and cancer. Only a small proportion of cigarette smokers develop lung cancer, but almost all people who develop lung cancer have been cigarette smokers. Similarly, although most people experiencing a severely threatening life event will not develop a depressive episode, Brown and Harris (1986) report that over 75% of depressions in the general community are brought on by a severely threatening event or major life difficulties. In each case the correlation will be low due to the large group not displaying the illness; but this obscures what is actually a very potent and robust relationship.

## Macrosocial and Cultural Models of Depression

It has been usual for psychiatrists and psychologists to ignore the impact of cultural factors in the development and transmission of depression.

Indeed, virtually all the research considered by us thus far represents expression of depression in European and North American populations during the past two decades. This ahistorical and culture-bound approach can lend itself to overconfident assertions about the ability of biological and individual variables to adequately explain the pathogenesis of depression. In particular, when there is relatively little variability in societal variables, their impact should be difficult to detect. However, cross-cultural and longitudinal research can increase our ability to detect societal changes and thus begin to illuminate the role of societywide changes in bringing about changes in rates of depression. Given what appears to be an increasing rate of depression in Western countries (Hagnell, Lanke, Rorsman, & Ojesjo, 1982; Weismann, 1987), it is perhaps time to go beyond genetic and psychological models to examine the data implicating broader societal variables in the etiology of depression.

In an illuminating beginning to such an effort, Kleinman (1988) presented several studies that should influence our view of depression. First, it appears that when nonindustrialized countries are compared with industrialized countries for rates of depression, the nonindustrialized countries show much greater variability, with particularly high rates being reported in a recent Ugandan study (Orley & Wing, 1979). In this study of Uganda, 14.4% of the men and 22.6% of the women were depressed. These point prevalence rates are three to five times higher than those for the United States. The comparatively high rates of depression were presumed to be a function of the general political unrest in Uganda. Also interesting in this vein is a report by Lin (1969; as cited in Kleinman, 1988) on changes in rates of depression in Taiwan over a 15-year period, using the same research team and research protocol in both assessments. The rates of depression were found to rise substantially during the period of Taiwan's modernization. Further, migrant workers, refugees, and immigrants are known to have higher rates of depression than the norm (Beiser, 1985; Beiser & Fleming, 1986). Finally, rates of suicide and presumed depression are known to vary with economic recessions and depressions (Hawton, 1986). In brief, rates of depression do vary at least in part with social and political conditions, and these macrosocial variables may elevate the size of the population at risk for depression. It is not clear from the data whether these macrosocial variables exert their influence by raising background stress, increasing the likelihood of severely threatening events, fostering dysfunctional thinking, or making coping more difficult, or whether they exert their influence through some alternative mechanism to those already discussed. Likewise, the factors accounting for the increasing rates of depression among U.S. young adults are not yet clear, but increases in divorce rates, sex-role strain and conflict, pressure on young people to specialize in a vocational/professional sense, and rates of the population below the poverty level are presumed to have some influence on these increasing rates (Beach & Nelson, 1990; Kleinman, 1988; Hafner, 1986).

## Conclusions

Two biological models of depression were reviewed, with a focus on the primary sources of data supporting these models. Both the genetic model and the biochemical (neurohormonal and neurotransmitter) models have stimulated considerable research. In hospitalized unipolar depressed populations and in bipolar depressed populations evidence supporting a genetic model has been forthcoming. Unfortunately, little work is currently available that adequately examines the role of genetic factors in the etiology of mild to moderate unipolar depression, the most commonly presented forms of depression. However, the work that is available suggests that a genetic diathesis is likely to be relevant in cases of severe depression.

The work on biochemistry in depression is currently in a state of flux. Biochemical abnormalities appear to be concomitants of depression rather than stable characteristics that precede and produce subsequent depression. Thus, while biochemical abnormalities may have a role in maintaining an ongoing episode of depression or mediating various symptoms of depression, it is not clear that they play a prominent early role in the chain of events leading to depression.

Six cognitive-behavioral theories of depression were reviewed, with a focus on the central themes that characterize those theories, namely, (1) cognitive distortions and negative self-schemata, (2) negative attributions, (3) reinforcement, (4) script disruption and self-focus, (5) self-control, and (6) problem solving and coping. Each of these theories has some empirical support based on correlational data. Interestingly, however, evidence is just beginning to accumulate from longitudinal research to support the etiological role of cognitive factors in depression. As with the biochemical factors studied in depression, cognitive-behavioral factors are, at a minimum, concomitants of depression. While they are clearly important in the maintenance of ongoing episodes of depression and appear to mediate many important symptoms in depression, it is not yet clear to what extent cognitive-behavioral factors play a prominent role early in the chain of events leading to nosological depression.

Interpersonal factors in depression, such as anger turned inward and marital discord, were also reviewed as factors contributing to depression. While the initial research on anger in depression has been questioned, the role of anger in the interaction of depressives and their partners has recently received significant attention. Social support within and outside the marriage appears to provide an important buffer against depression, but it is the provision of support by close others that emerges as most protective against depression. Finally, the role of marital discord as a correlate of depression is very clear, and the role of marital discord as a precipitant and/or maintainer of depression is becoming increasingly evident. In addition, stress research has shown that negative life events in marriage, such as separation and marital arguments, play an important etiological role in depression.

Taken as a whole the evidence available to date suggests that marital discord is implicated as a major stressor and as an important aspect of support and coping processes. Marital discord may well be one of the most potent variables among those implicated in the production and maintenance of depression. When it is present in the context of depression, it seems likely to be worthy of therapeutic attention. Accordingly, in the next chapter we will present a marital discord model of depression. Following our presentation of the marital discord model of depression, we will outline a marital treatment program for depression that has proven successful in alleviating both depression and marital discord (Beach & O'Leary, 1986; O'Leary & Beach, 1990).

# 3

## The Marital Discord Model of Depression

For the maritally discordant individual, the marital relationship may play a powerful role in the development and maintenance of depression as well as having potential utility in promoting recovery and maintenance of gains. The marital situation holds, at a minimum, considerable influence over feelings of well-being (cf. Diener, 1984) and may often play a central role in the etiology and maintenance of the depressive episode (cf. Beach & Nelson, 1990). The marital discord model of depression is designed to help focus available research on the task confronting the clinician by identifying an integrated set of "points of intervention" to guide clinical activity. To the extent it achieves this goal, it will help organize clinical activity in a natural and fluid manner, allowing the clinician to tailor interventions to fit the couple while simultaneously remaining focused on those targets of therapy that are held to produce positive outcome (Beach & Bauserman, 1990).

Following an account of the evolution of the marital discord model of depression, we present an elaborated model of the relationship between marital discord and depression. We identify six facets of the marital relationship that are capable of providing social support and enhanced coping and five facets of the marital relationship capable of inducing considerable stress and strain. We also examine the role of depression in further aggravating ongoing marital discord, the role of cognition in the marital model of depression, and approaches to integrating the marital model of depression with other models discussed in Chapter 2. An overview of the basic model can be seen in Figure 3-1.

As can be seen, the marital relationship areas of relevance to support and coping are couple cohesion, acceptance and encouragement of emotional expression, coping assistance, direct self-esteem support, percep-

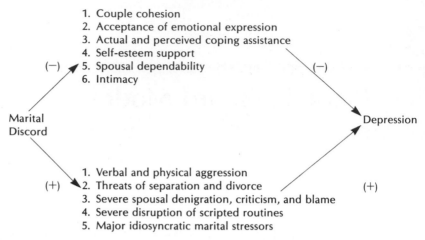

1. Couple cohesion
2. Acceptance of emotional expression
3. Actual and perceived coping assistance
4. Self-esteem support
5. Spousal dependability
6. Intimacy

(−)                                                (−)

Marital
Discord                                                Depression

(+)                                                (+)

1. Verbal and physical aggression
2. Threats of separation and divorce
3. Severe spousal denigration, criticism, and blame
4. Severe disruption of scripted routines
5. Major idiosyncratic marital stressors

FIGURE 3-1. A marital discord model of depression.

tion of spousal dependability and enduring commitment to the relationship, and the presence of a confiding and intimate relationship. Marital discord is shown to decrease (−) available support from the partner. On the negative, stress-enhancing side are the marital relationship areas of overt hostility, threats of divorce, severe denigration, severe disruption of scripted marital routines, and other major idiosyncratic stressors identified by the couple. Marital discord is shown to increase (+) levels of major stressors in the marital relationship. Taken together, the decrease in marital support and increase in marital stress are shown to mediate the relationship of marital discord to depression. Each area represents a relatively distinct facet of marital interaction that has shown some evidence of being related to depressive symptomatology and can be a direct focus of attention in marital therapy.

## Development and Empirical Background of the Model

We begin by providing a brief developmental account of our attempts to understand the relationship between marital discord and depression. This account helps highlight possible limitations on the generalizability of our current model. In particular, it will become clear that our model may be generalized most easily to outpatient treatment settings serving mildly to moderately depressed wives who admit being in moderately to severely discordant marriages. The model may well be generalizable far beyond the context and population with which we have worked. However, it is often helpful to the practicing clinician to know which parameters have already been tested by the authors and which remain to be explored.

Interest in the use of marital therapy for depression at the State University of New York at Stony Brook predates our explicit focus on diagnosed depression; it has its roots in uncontrolled clinical observation of couples presenting for marital therapy at the university's Marital Therapy Clinic as well as in observations made during an early marital therapy outcome study conducted there (Turkewitz & O'Leary, 1981). It was observed clinically that many couples presenting for marital therapy were displaying high levels of depressive symptomatology. Usually it was the wife who appeared most depressed, but sometimes husbands were more depressed and sometimes both spouses seemed depressed. When a widely used measure of depression was used to screen all couples presenting for marital therapy, it was found that mild to moderate levels of depressive symptomatology were present in over 50% of the cases (cf. Beach et al., 1985). In addition, the therapists working in the clinic noticed that these "depressed" couples were getting better in marital therapy (cf. Jacobson, Follette, & Pagel, 1986). As their marriages improved, their moods seemed to improve as well.

Depressed wives seeking marital therapy at the marital clinic would often describe a history of seeking help from physicians or other primary health care providers in the community. The wives typically believed that their symptoms of depression were related to their ongoing marital discord, but they had either been unwilling to discuss marital problems in detail or their physicians had been reluctant to discuss these issues with them. While in some cases this initial help seeking led to referral for marital therapy or advice about marital difficulties, more commonly the result was the prescription of antidepressants or anxiolytics to help with sleep or mood. Most typically, wives reported that the pharmacological interventions produced only small initial beneficial effects on mood, which were then followed by substantial residual symptoms and rapid relapse (cf. Rounsaville et al., 1979a).

It was only a short time after these initial observations that Weissman (1979) called for greater attention to marital relationships as a possible target of intervention with depressed patients. Concurrently, Ilfeld (1977) published data indicating that stress in the family demonstrated a strong relationship to depressive symptomatology, and Brown and Harris (1978) published their seminal work on the link between a supportive, confiding relationship and protection against the development of depression. Meanwhile in sociological circles, the importance of social support and primary relationships had been under discussion for some time (cf. Caplan, 1974; Weiss, 1974). Taken together, these various threads of research and clinical observation made a compelling case that marital therapy could be the therapy of choice for the type of depressed patients we were used to seeing—explicitly discordant couples who wanted to improve their marital relationships and who suffered with the concurrent problem of one or both spouses meeting diagnostic criteria for depression. Inspired in this manner, it was decided that initial trials of marital therapy for depression should be undertaken (Beach & O'Leary, 1986).

Even though we had already worked successfully with discordant couples in which one member appeared depressed, and despite the knowledge that other marital therapists had successfully worked with depressed, discordant clients using approaches similar to our own (Jacobson & Margolin, 1979), we wondered about the ethics of proposing marital therapy as a treatment for depression. Good individually oriented treatments for depression were already available (Beck, Rush, Shaw, & Emery, 1979; Klerman et al., 1984), and marital therapy was a relative unknown. In addition, the effectiveness of pharmacological interventions for depression seemed well established. However, the evidence was strong that individual and somatic interventions for depression seemed to do little to routinely improve discordant relationships (Beach, Winters, & Weintraub, 1986; Bothwell & Weissman, 1977; DiMascio et al., 1979; Friedman, 1975). If the marital relationship enhancement requested by discordant, depressed couples was to be forthcoming, then, it would have to be through some intervention targeted directly at the marital relationship. Thus, at least for the group of explicitly discordant, depressed couples, trials of marital therapy seemed ethically permissible.

Another reason to pursue trials of marital therapy for depression was to address the very clear suffering produced by unresolved marital discord and to highlight the reality of this problem. Indeed, the great hardships imposed by the occurrence of marital discord in the context of depression were not widely appreciated by many of the professionals responsible for supervising the recovery process in depression. Thus many psychologists and psychiatrists neither assessed nor were concerned to treat the marital or family context of the depression, even when it was quite obviously disturbed. Consideration of the greatly underappreciated impact of marital discord added to our conviction that trials of marital therapy in the treatment of depression were ethically warranted.

Thus the marital discord model of depression that has evolved at Stony Brook was formed in the course of working with maritally discordant couples. Since it was developed in the context of couples who presented themselves for treatment as a couple to a marital therapy clinic, its focus has always been on explicitly maritally discordant couples who presented themselves as having marital difficulties they wished to resolve. In this context, at least one of the partners, and typically both, had some degree of commitment to their relationship and some desire to improve their marriage. Accordingly, the clinical experiences that inform our approach to treatment may not be directly applicable to couples in which one spouse has already decided (firmly) to leave the relationship, cases in which one spouse refuses to come to the clinic for therapy, or those couples who deny marital discord. However, within the context of therapy involving explicitly discordant couples who are both available for therapy, the marital discord model of depression fits nicely with our own clinical experience, and we have found it helpful in guiding the treatment of depression occurring in the context of marital discord (Beach & O'Leary, 1986; O'Leary & Beach, 1990).

## Initial Conceptual Concerns

Having decided that a marital intervention for depression was called for, we knew that two issues required attention. First, perhaps the marital problems characterizing depressed, discordant couples would turn out to be substantially different from the problems of other discordant couples. If so, this would suggest a substantial discontinuity between the problems recorded in the basic literature on marital discord and those of the depressed, discordant couples we were trying to understand. In the most extreme case, it could suggest that the treatment packages and techniques shown to be effective with other maritally discordant couples might have little applicability to alleviating marital discord in a depressed population. The second concern was over the possibility that all depressed patients might be maritally dysfunctional, even those scoring in the nondiscordant range on standard self-report inventories. If this were true, it would suggest that providing marital therapy only to couples with overt marital discord would be overrestrictive. Perhaps it would be discovered that *all* married depressed persons were in need of some form of marital therapy.

These issues represent ongoing areas of concern and have not yet been fully resolved. However, there is sufficient empirical work to provide the outline of an answer to each question. To address the first issue (i.e., whether the marital discord experienced by depressed persons is qualitatively different from that commonly encountered in marital therapy clinics and studied by marital researchers), we review the evidence on the nature of marital relationships among the discordant depressed. We address the second concern (i.e., whether apparently nondiscordant depressed couples are really discordant) by examining data on interactional differences between depressed couples who report themselves to be discordant and depressed couples who report themselves to be nondiscordant.

## Marital Discord in the Context of Depression

Descriptions of the discordant, depressed dyad are not frequent in the literature. Nevertheless, sufficient work has accumulated to allow comment on four major areas of interactional problems among the discordant depressed. First, as might be anticipated, depressed patients engage in more "depressive" behaviors in interacting with their spouses than do other types of spouses. Interestingly, it may also be true that they engage in these depressive behaviors more with intimates than with strangers. Second, discordant, depressed couples show less cohesion in their relationships than do other couples. This lack of cohesion appears to be particularly evident when one spouse is not depressed, but it may be attenuated when both spouses are depressed. Third, it appears that there may be more asymmetry in the relationships of depressed, discordant dyads. In particular, depressed persons may be more likely to assume a passive position and let decision making be done for them. Fourth, as is the case in other discordant relationships, there is considerable anger openly expressed in the interactions of depressed, discordant couples as well as anger that is felt but not expressed. We examine each of these findings briefly below.

### DEPRESSIVE BEHAVIOR

The nature of prototypically depressive interactive behavior has been highlighted and substantially clarified by the research team at the Oregon Research Institute (Biglan et al., 1985; Hops et al., 1987). They define the category of depressive (or distressed) behaviors to include behaviors such as self-derogation, physical and psychological complaints, and displays of depressed affect. These categories are useful both for the conceptual clarification they provide and for their direct clinical descriptive utility. For example, in research done by Hautzinger, Linden, and Hoffman (1982; Linden, Hautzinger, & Hoffman, 1983), it was found that discordant, depressed members of a dyad made more statements reflecting negative well-being, more negative statements about themselves, and more negative statements about their future expectations than did their nondepressed spouses, as well as more such statements than did the nondepressed, discordant comparison couples. While not identified by Hautzinger and colleagues (1982) as "depressive," these behaviors clearly fit in this category as defined by the Oregon group. Importantly, Hautzinger and colleagues (1982) contrasted their depressed, discordant group with a nondepressed, discordant group. Thus these "depressive" behaviors could be shown to be unique to the depressed patients and not simply a function of marital discord.

Similarly, Beach and Nelson (1989) examined the problem-solving interactions of depressed, discordant couples and contrasted their behavior with that of nondepressed, discordant couples. Although using a different coding system, the study again found that "depressive" behaviors as defined by the Oregon group occurred much more often in the depressed, discordant group than in the nondepressed, discordant group. In addition, the very high rates were confined to the identified patient. Interestingly, these "depressive" behaviors also appeared to have a suppressive effect on spousal aggression, as predicted both by the coercion model (Biglan et al., 1988) and by Coyne's (1976) interpersonal model of depression (see Chapter 2 for more information on each model), and this suppressive effect appeared to wear off as the duration of the marital discord increased (Nelson & Beach, in press). However, nondepressed dyads demonstrated the suppression effect to a nonsignificantly greater degree than the depressed couples (Nelson & Beach, in press). Thus "depressive" behavior appears to be integrally related to the overall functioning of maritally discordant, depressed couples as well as to the functioning of discordant couples in general. Depressed spouses are unique only in their very high rates of depressive behavior. In a related note, Hinchliffe, Hooper, and Roberts (1978) report that depressed patients appeared to become substantially less negative and "pathological" in their behavior when interacting with strangers, underscoring the possibility that much "depressive" behavior is spouse-specific.

Figuring prominently in the Oregon group's analysis of depressive behavior is display of depressed affect, including slow speech, disturbance of speech, tearfulness, sighs, looking away, whining, and sad facial expression. Recent evidence suggests that increased frequency and latency of pauses in speaking may be characteristic of depressed persons in any task focusing on personal issues (Siegman, 1987) and that decreases in pausing time and increases in eye contact during discussions may predict ultimate positive response to somatic treatment (cf. Ellgring, Wagner, & Clarke, 1980; Greden & Carroll, 1980). Thus observable changes in rates of "depressive" behaviors may be of value as early predictors of clinical response, as well as being of interest due to their effects on the spouse.

Given the intuitive appeal of the Oregon group's proposal that depressed patients will display elevated rates of prototypically "depressive" behavior in interactions involving the spouse or family members and the strong corroboration already forthcoming, it seems reasonable to conclude that this type of behavior is likely to be seen often by marital therapists working with depressed, discordant couples. In addition, given its direct influence on the partner, it may sometimes need to be a direct target of intervention. Given their high rate of occurrence and their particular prominence in interactions with the spouse, depressive behaviors clearly can change the affective tone of marital therapy. Accordingly, the need for ways of responding to "depressive venting" in session represents one way in which marital therapy for depression differs from standard marital therapy.

## MARITAL COHESION

A second area that has received some empirical attention is that of marital and family cohesion. In a direct investigation of the relationship between marital cohesion and level of depression, Beach, Nelson, and O'Leary (1988) contrasted depressed, discordant with nondepressed, discordant and community wives. While substantial similarity was found between the two discordant groups on most marital measures, they were found to differ significantly on the dyadic cohesion subscale of the Dyadic Adjustment Scale (DAS; Spanier, 1976). In addition, group differences in dyadic cohesion accounted for unique variance in depression beyond that which could be accounted for by cognitive style differences between the two groups. Thus level of cohesion in the marriage emerged as an important variable differentiating the marital relationships of discordant, depressed and discordant, nondepressed wives. In a similar vein, Billings and Moos (1982) found that adults who were in families low in cohesion were higher in depressive symptomatology and, Monroe and colleagues (1986) found that the cohesion subscale of the DAS predicted subsequent symptoms of depression.

These results are consistent with our clinical observations regarding discordant, depressed couples. They most typically are feeling very distant and isolated from each other. We have come to anticipate that building time for the couple to be together on a regular, predictable basis in a hedonically positive atmosphere will be required early in therapy. Among couples in which the husband is also depressed, we have found some couples who report spending sufficient time together. In these cases the problem has been that time together was experienced as being stifling, boring, or hedonically negative. Thus couples in which both partners are depressed still require considerable attention to the enhancement of couple cohesion (i.e., shared positive activities).

In sum, the results obtained to date suggest that the depressed, discordant sample may be skewed in the direction of low cohesion. This observation has led us to put great emphasis on the development of cohesion in the dyad as an important early component of marital therapy for depression. In particular, we tend to avoid contracting approaches and focus instead on enhancing caring gestures and pleasant interaction.

Indeed, even problem-solving training is commonly introduced as a way for the couple to gain more experience in expressing ideas and working together cohesively as a team. The idea of making the problem-solving process as hedonically positive as possible, with as much display of caring as possible—even if this slows the problem-solving process itself—flows from our increased emphasis on enhancing cohesion. Again, this represents a shift but not a departure from standard marital therapy interventions.

## ASYMMETRY

A third area that has received some empirical attention is apparent lack of symmetry in the interactions of depressed persons and their spouses. In the study by Hautzinger and colleagues (1982) discussed above, the authors also noted that depressed persons evaluated themselves negatively but did not evaluate their spouses negatively. Conversely, their spouses rarely mentioned their own well-being but evaluated the depressed partner negatively. Interestingly, they found that spouses of depressed patients seldom agreed with their partners' statements, and though they offered help, they did so with concurrent negative verbalizations. It appears that discussions in Hautzinger and colleagues' (1982) study were dominated by verbalizations about the depressed patient's negative well-being, with both participants focusing on the depressed patient. The high rate of depressive behavior on the part of the depressed patient appears to focus both partners' verbalizations on the depressed spouse's feelings and symptoms of depression as a convenient alternative to discussion of marital problems.

Work by Merikangas, Ranelli, and Kupfer (1979) further supports the hypothesis of asymmetry in the interactions of depressed, discordant couples. They found that when female inpatients were depressed, they showed a very strong tendency to change their opinions regarding revealed-differences tasks and make them more similar to those of their partners following discussion. However, as their depression lifted, the balance of who changed their opinion became more even between the two partners. At a minimum, it appears that ongoing depression occurring in the context of marital discord disposes the depressed partner to be less confident in an assertive or combative role, contributing to various asymmetries in the couple's interaction. Thus depressed couples should show less prolonged "battling" interactions and more interactions characterized by brief hostile exchanges followed by withdrawal. Also, the characteristic signature of the depressed and discordant couple is that it is difficult for them to overcome the avoidance (cf. Mitchell, Cronkite, &

Moos, 1983) and withdrawal that typically follows their hostile exchanges. Clinically, we have seen spouses who would avoid all interaction with each other for several days following a rather minor argument. Accordingly, it is likely to be necessary to enhance spouse-specific assertion during the course of therapy if couple issues are to be resolved. Dealing with these enhanced avoidance tendencies of depressed, discordant couples calls for a somewhat different emphasis in therapy and requires considerable skill in terms of keeping the process of therapy on track.

## OVERT HOSTILITY

Finally, a fourth area receiving empirical attention is the presence of overtly hostile and aggressive behavior in the depressed, discordant dyad. Several studies have shown that spouses of depressed persons may feel quite hostile following marital interactions (Kahn, Coyne, & Margolin, 1985; Arkowitz, Holliday, & Hutter, 1982), even though attempts are made to suppress the direct expression of the hostile feelings. Likewise, several studies have shown that both partners within the depressed, discordant dyad are likely to engage in aggressive behavior (Biglan et al., 1985; Hooley & Hahlweg, 1985; Beach & Nelson, 1989), including mutual criticism and reciprocation of negative partner behavior. However, high rates of depressive behavior may partially suppress the expression of considerable hostility by the spouse (Biglan et al., 1985). Similarly, the avoidance patterns adopted by depressed spouses may lead them to suppress the expression of much of their own hostility. If the tendency to completely suppress the expression of feelings is allowed to continue in therapy, this will undermine the ability of therapy to bring about real and lasting changes in the relationship. Thus marital therapists working with depressed, discordant couples may need to be especially alert to subtle cues that the whole story is not being told or that spouses are not really leveling with each other. At the same time, marital therapists must be particularly aware of the likely destructive consequences of allowing spouses to express their hostile feelings in an unmodulated manner.

## CONCLUSIONS

Taken together, the evidence reviewed above suggests that the depressed and discordant couple can be quite challenging. They are in need of a therapeutic approach for their marital problems that can help them connect with each other and build positive time together, talk openly and directly with each other, reverse the pattern of stifling honest interaction, and develop an egalitarian method of resolving marital problems. Dealing with these needs requires some modification of standard marital therapy packages. However, the evidence also suggests that depressed, discordant couples engage in many of the same behaviors as other discordant couples (cf. Gotlib & Whiffen, 1989; Hooley, 1986; Nelson & Beach, in press). Accordingly, much of marital therapy as it has been practiced with maritally discordant couples in general is likely to be applicable, with appropriate modifications, to the depressed, discordant couple.

In some respects it should come as no surprise that there are many commonalities between depressed, discordant couples and their nondepressed counterparts. It is likely that many of the couples considered by marital researchers to be discordant (i.e., those presenting for marital therapy) actually included a depressed member (Beach et al., 1985). In addition, marital discord seems to precede depression, suggesting that most discordant, depressed couples spend considerable time being simply discordant before one spouse succumbs to depression. Accordingly, it seems reasonable to expect that many of the techniques available for working with maritally discordant couples should be applicable, with appropriate changes, to depressed, discordant couples.

## Are All Depressed Couples Discordant?

The literature clearly suggests that explicitly discordant couples in which one member is depressed look a great deal like other explicitly discordant couples. But what of depressed couples who report themselves to be relatively nondiscordant? If these couples with a depressed member are also really discordant, then perhaps they need to receive some sort of marital therapy as well. Of course, for these couples one might expect that marital therapy would have to be framed somewhat differently and that there would be some initial reluctance to focus on relationship work. Nevertheless, if these couples are truly discordant, it is likely that resolving their discord would be a necessary component of any program hoping to produce sustained recovery. While relatively little work to date has adequately addressed this issue, it is interesting that the evidence to date does *not* support the position that depressed couples who report satisfactory marriages have seemingly discordant interactions or are likely to benefit from marital therapy.

Nondiscordant, depressed couples do not show prototypically discordant, negative interactional patterns (Biglan et al., 1985; Hooley,

1986); the interaction of these couples appears to be quite different from that of their explicitly discordant counterparts. Furthermore, the available evidence, although limited, suggests that marital intervention with couples who deny marital problems is unlikely to be very helpful to them (Whisman, Jacobson, Fruzzetti, & Schmaling, 1988). Thus at present there is no reason to routinely consider marital therapy for depressed persons in the absence of evidence of problems in the marriage.

Clinical reports persist, however, of cases in which a spouse or an entire family had adapted to one person's depression and subsequently experienced difficulty with that person's symptomatic improvement. Likewise, clinical reports suggest the possibility that in some cases depression may mask severe marital discord until symptomatic improvement brings the problems into the open (normally as the formerly depressed spouse becomes more assertive). Our own findings do not suggest that this is always or even typically the case for mildly maritally discordant couples receiving individual therapy. Indeed, even for moderately maritally discordant couples we found that it was as likely for the relationship to improve somewhat as it was for the relationship to deteriorate for wives receiving cognitive therapy. Further, in a more mildly discordant sample than our own, the tendency was for cognitive therapy to be associated with some improvement in the marital relationship on average (Whisman et al., 1988). Thus while the search for reliable indications of "hidden" marital pathology in depressed, nondiscordant couples should probably be continued, and clinicians should not be too surprised if on occasion marital therapy is found to be necessary for a case that initially presented as depressed but nondiscordant, it is inappropriate, given the current evidence, to recommend marital work as a treatment for depression in the absence of overt marital discord.

## Conclusions

The preliminary findings available to date require replication and a continued search for behaviors most characteristic of the depressed, discordant couple. Already, however, we have an outline of the many similarities as well as differences between discordant couples in which one spouse is depressed and discordant couples in which neither partner is depressed. The outline to date provides encouragement for making modifications in standard marital therapy treatment packages to focus attention on the areas most in need of work for depressed and discordant couples. However, it is clear that there is no need to abandon the basic literature on marital discord or create an entirely new approach to marital therapy. On many measures, both self-report and observational, the population of depressed, discordant couples overlaps substantially with the population of nondepressed, discordant couples. This suggests the happy conclusion that marital patterns that have been carefully explicated in the basic literature on marital discord are likely to obtain in large part for depressed, discordant couples as well. In addition, it suggests that prior to becoming depressed, the discordant and depressed couples may have been very much like other discordant couples. Accordingly, the basic literature on marital discord should be very informative in trying to better understand the development of depression in the context of marital discord.

## Basic Literature on Marital Discord: Implications for Depression

The empirical base for understanding the development and maintenance of marital discord has continued to expand rapidly (Weiss & Heyman, 1990). While we will not attempt to provide a comprehensive review of this work, we will briefly summarize the most clinically relevant aspects of the basic work.

As couples become discordant, they find the balance of events in their relationship changing in a negative direction (Barnett & Nietzel, 1979; Birchler, Weiss, & Vincent, 1975; Margolin, 1981). They become more reactive to negative behaviors from their spouse, exaggerating the stress engendered by negative exchanges (Levenson & Gottman, 1983; Jacobson, Waldron, & Moore, 1980; Jacobson, Follette, & McDonald, 1982). They begin to more readily reciprocate negatives from their spouse (Billings, 1979; Gottman, 1979; Margolin & Wampold, 1981; Revenstorf, Hahlweg, Schindler, & Vogel, 1984; Vivian, Smith, & O'Leary, 1988). Discordant wives may fail to edit their partners' negative behavior (Notarius, Benson, Sloane, Vanzetti, & Hornyak, 1989), leading them to respond with increasingly high rates of negative behavior; both spouses may perceive each other's behavior as more negative (Floyd & Markman, 1983), more blameworthy, and more deserving of punishment (Fincham et al., 1987). In conjunction with this increase in frequency and perceived negativity of marital exchanges between spouses, discordant spouses are also more confident than their nondiscordant counterparts that their negative judgments of their spouse are true (Noller & Venardos, 1986). These changes result in considerable difficulty in attempting to communicate about or resolve existing problems (Gottman, Markman, & Notarius, 1977; Koren, Carlton, & Shaw, 1980), generating considerable frustration for the discordant couple. This increasing frustration is likely to be manifested in higher rates of criticism, demands, or nagging on the part of one spouse, and withdrawal, avoidance, and hurt feelings on the part of the other spouse (Christensen, 1987). In short, the spouses often find themselves in a "coercive spiral" (Patterson & Reid, 1970; Weiss, Hops, & Patterson, 1973) in which each partner tries to influence the other in an escalating exchange of negative behavior.

As we thought about this common scenario, we were struck by two major points of relevance for depression. First, in accord with Epstein (1985), we were impressed by the direct correspondence between common facets of marital discord and the symptoms of depression. Feeling discouraged about the future, feeling that one is being punished, feeling disappointed in oneself, and experiencing loss of interest in significant others occur both in depression and in marital discord uncomplicated by depression. In marital discord uncomplicated by depression, these feelings and beliefs are confined to relationship-specific areas. But simply by virtue of being maritally discordant, individuals may be viewed as having "a head start" on meeting criteria for depression. If these thoughts and feelings begin to generalize, the maritally discordant individual will quickly appear to be depressed. In addition, feelings of hopelessness about the future of the marriage and one's ability to resolve marital problems are quite common among the maritally discordant. In combination with initially low self-esteem or strong dependency needs, one might expect these feelings of hopelessness to generalize rapidly to other areas, precipitating a depressive episode.

Second, we were impressed by the extreme stress, loss of social support, and ineffective coping that occurred in situations of marital discord. Indeed, it was often the sense of isolation, the chronic daily stress engendered by marital problems, and the perception that nothing could be done to bring relief that were the focus of complaints by depressed, discordant couples. For spouses who are not yet depressed, the loss of support and increased level of chronic stress involved in marital discord should be expected to push them in the direction of an episode of depression. For spouses who are already depressed, the lack of support and ongoing stress of marital discord should be expected to intensify their dysphoria and confirm their sense of hopelessness and isolation. Even for spouses who are well along in the process of recovering from depression, the lack of social support and ongoing stress of marital discord should be expected to hold them back from experiencing full recovery. Thus the stress and loss of social support inherent in marital discord are critical areas to elaborate in a marital discord model of depression. In addition, any effective marital therapy program should reduce the couple's sense of hopelessness about ever coping effectively with their marital problems.

## An Elaborated Marital Discord Model of Depression

We had evidence that marital discord was linked to depression, and we had good evidence that there were effective treatment packages for improving the marriages of discordant couples (Beach & O'Leary, 1985; Weiss & Heyman, 1990). Why not simply have a model with one point of intervention—marital discord—and identify the treatment packages most effective for alleviating marital discord? This is not an entirely unreasonable proposal and in many respects represents our initial logic in attempting to work with discordant, depressed couples. However, it ultimately must be considered unsatisfactory. First, it does little to highlight areas likely to be in need of more attention in a depressed sample; that is, even if marital discord in the context of depression is similar to marital discord in other contexts, there may be certain aspects of the relationship that are more intimately related than others to the production of depressive symptomatology. An elaborated model can draw attention to those areas most in need of attention when the aim is to decrease depressive symptomatology.

A second reason for elaborating the model is that particular treatment packages are too tied to the technology of the present. Clearly, new forms of marital therapy are being developed and tested (Beach & Bauserman, 1990). An elaborated model is more likely to be able to incorporate new technologies as they become available than is a rote application of an omnibus treatment package. In addition, an application of a treatment package does not represent the reality of clinical practice. An elaborated model is better able to guide the clinician in the flexible manner necessitated by the idiosyncrasies of clients' particular problems. Thus an elaborated model is better able to provide the experienced clinician with useful stimulation and guidance than is the specification of a particular treatment package. In a similar vein, there appears to be some benefit in allowing clinicians to use clinical judgment in applying marital therapy treatments in a more tailored form (Jacobson, Schmaling, Holtzworth-Munroe, et al., 1989), and an elaborated model provides guidance for this more exacting clinical activity. Accordingly, we began to search the literature and our own clinical experience for more specific points of intervention of relevance to depression occurring in the context of marital discord.

## Marital Discord and Loss of Social Support

As described in Chapter 2, the stress, social support, and coping models of depression have produced a veritable explosion of research and literature reviews in recent years (cf. Goldberger & Breznitz, 1982; Hobfall, 1986; Lin, Dean, & Ensel, 1986). However, clearer theoretical formulations of the nature of social support and basic empirical work testing these propositions continue to be worked out (cf. Fisher & Reason, 1988). Several facets of social support appear to be of most relevance when considering the marriage and its role in the formation of depressive symptomatology. In particular, we see six facets of social support both as being conceptually distinct from one another and as having received empirical documentation with regard to their relevance for depression. It seems likely that this list will be further refined and elaborated in the future, but in each case, clear relevance for processes occurring within the marital dyad is present. The six facets of social support we highlight below are: (1) couple cohesion, (2) acceptance of emotional expression, (3) actual and perceived coping assistance, (4) self-esteem support, (5) spousal dependability, and (6) intimacy and confiding.


## COUPLE COHESION

Couple cohesion within marriage can be defined most simply as the amount of positive time a couple spends together engaging in joint, pleasant activities. Cohesion has been referred to as "companionship" (Rook, 1987), "cohesion" (Spanier, 1976), or simply "social support" (Monroe et al., 1986). As might be expected, both men and women place considerable value on cohesion in marital relationships (Cochran & Peplau, 1985). Indeed, its absence is a frequent source of marital dissatisfaction (Wills, Weiss, & Patterson, 1974) and is related to increasing demoralization (Schaefer & Burnett, 1987) and depressive symptomatology over time (Beach, Arias, & O'Leary, 1988; Monroe et al., 1986). Beach and Tesser (1987) hypothesized that high levels of cohesion in marriage may also buffer stress. The spouse is the individual typically seen as providing the most opportunities for closeness, ability to be oneself, social interaction, and shared interests, making marriage a particularly salient relationship with regard to opportunities for cohesion (Denoff, 1982). It appears, then, that cohesion is a central aspect of marital interaction and may be a central aspect of the dyad's protection against depressive symptomatology. Thus the enhancement of cohesion in the dyad would appear to be an obvious point of intervention with discordant, depressed couples.

Cohesive behaviors include common, everyday interactional events, such as simple displays of affection, shared positive time together, making time to be together for such routine enjoyable activities as meal time or other shared family time, or routine discussions of the day or joint projects. These behaviors constitute a great reservoir of stability, familiarity, and hedonically positive experience. The familiarity and positive quality of these interactions would be expected to be a powerful reassurance that things are not really as unsettled and unpredictable as they might otherwise seem in the face of problems arising external to the marital relationship. In addition, cohesive activities would be expected to provide reassurance that occasional arguments or strained interactions with the spouse are not as serious as they might otherwise seem. Finally, cohesive activities provide good distraction from worry and self-focused concern, along with an opportunity for relaxation. Thus "cohesive" events should be well suited to serve as "stress opposing experiences" (Cochrane, 1988).

## ACCEPTANCE OF EMOTIONAL EXPRESSION

A second element of social support that has been discussed in the literature is the opportunity to express one's feelings and to feel understood and accepted by another (Lehman, Ellard, & Wortman, 1986). Indeed, Sarason, Shearin, Pierce, and Sarason (1987) suggest that being involved in a relationship that yields a sense of acceptance and being loved may be the most central component of effective social support. It is disclosure of *feelings* to one's partner, rather than disclosure of facts, that appears to be related most strongly to marital satisfaction (Hendrick, 1981), and it is likely that it is the perception that one's spouse will be accepting of disclosure of one's feelings that is most related to feeling understood and accepted.

The spouse is the individual most likely to be turned to for expression of feelings and support in time of trouble (Lieberman, 1982) as well as the person who typically provides the most opportunities to discuss personal problems and feelings in general (Denoff, 1982). Thus, in a relationship in which one spouse rejects the other's direct expression of feelings, there could be a loss of social support that would be difficult to replace via other relationships. Similarly, where one spouse attempts to "cheer up" the partner by denying his/her feelings of depression, one might anticipate a worsening of symptoms rather than an improvement (cf. Wortman, 1984). Conversely, in any relationship, taking the perspective of the other and accepting the other's expression of feelings through reflection and accurate empathy is useful in offering comfort (Burleson & Samter, 1985; Young, Giles, & Plantz, 1982). Thus when spouses are able to be appropriately empathic they may provide optimal support. Interestingly, the opportunity for emotional sharing may be more important to wives than to husbands (Parelman, 1982). Thus enhancement of husbands' acceptance of emotional expression by their wives may be particularly important when the wife is depressed.

Another mechanism that may link the presence of an accepting other with stress resilience and decreased dysphoria has been suggested by Pennebaker (1988). It appears that the act of telling another about a traumatic event can reduce stress. In particular, a marital environment that is high in acceptance of emotional expression may provide opportunities for spouses to reprocess in a calmer state the difficult or threatening situations they face. In addition to helping the stressed partner calm down and feel reassured for the moment, such expressions of thoughts and feelings appear to convey lasting benefits. Thus the marriage is likely to buffer stress and protect against depression more effectively if acceptance of emotional expression is high.

A history of acceptance of one's emotional disclosures would also be expected to enhance and encourage confiding. Particularly for a depressed and discordant couple, one might expect little risk taking and thus little confiding in the absence of high levels of acceptance of emotional expression. Thus therapeutic work aimed at enhancing acceptance of emotional expression may also be a necessary precursor to work aimed at increasing confiding and intimacy. The enhancement of confiding and intimacy is discussed below as a facet of social support protecting against depression in its own right.

## ACTUAL AND PERCEIVED COPING ASSISTANCE

A third aspect of social support likely to be important in buffering stress and protecting against depression is guidance (Weiss, 1974) or actual coping assistance offered by the spouse (cf. Thoits, 1986). If advice or aid from a spouse helps the depressed person deal with a disturbing situation, it should be expected that an enhanced sense of environmental mastery and control would result. This in turn would be expected to reduce experienced symptoms (cf. Abramson, Metalsky, & Alloy, 1989; Bandura, 1986; Brown, 1979; Brown & Harris, 1978; Pearlin, Lieberman, Menaghan, & Mullan, 1981). In addition, through offers of concrete aid, a spouse may help reduce the perceived threat of the stressor as his/her partner reappraises the level of threat (Lazarus, 1966, 1967). Thus concrete aid from the partner should buffer stressors arising outside the relationship. While some offers of concrete aid are likely to be unsolicited, it is likely that in many cases the offer of help will follow or grow out of successful couple problem solving. Thus joint problem solving and direct communication between spouses is likely to be necessary for concrete coping assistance to be forthcoming in the most helpful way.

Of particular importance in the context of marital discord, when the stressful situation to be dealt with is *in* the relationship, joint problem solving and offers of concrete aid may result in the direct and immediate alleviation of the stressor. Indeed, Pearlin and Schooler (1978) found that the ability to directly address problems appeared to reduce stress most effectively in the domain of marriage. Conversely, an inability to exert control over reducing conflict in the marriage appears to increase felt dissatisfaction (Madden & Janoff-Bulman, 1981). In a similar way, enhancement of joint problem solving is likely to reduce the extent to which the nondepressed spouse actively hinders the depressed spouse's attempts to achieve other important outcomes. Change in this domain should also decrease distress and increase well-being (Ruehlman & Wolchik, 1988). Thus, by helping couples address marital problems more directly in a joint problem-solving framework, there may be both direct and indirect benefits for the reduction of depressive symptomatology. Since depressed partners are particularly likely to avoid problems rather than directly confronting them (Mitchell et al., 1983), a direct problem-solving framework appears particularly well suited for increasing the concrete support available from the nondepressed spouse in the discordant couple.


## SELF-ESTEEM SUPPORT

A fourth facet of social support potentially applicable to the marital dyad has been referred to as "self-esteem support," "reassurance of worth" (Weiss, 1974), "affirmation" (Vanfossen, 1986), or simply "social support" (Brehm, 1984). It has been argued that esteem-enhancing support is very important for many types of health maintenance (Heller, Swindle, & Dusenbury, 1986). This type of support is generally considered to include behaviors relevant to appreciation, complimenting, and noticing positive traits in the partner. Interestingly, in a study conducted by Vanfossen (1986), it was the variable of affirmation that was most strongly and consistently related to well-being for wives. Receiving affirmation within the marital dyad was related to lower levels of depressive symptomatology, higher levels of self-esteem, and increased feelings of mastery. This type of support may be particularly important to wives, since they tend to be more self-critical on average than are husbands (Carver & Ganellen, 1983). It is also more common for wives to feel unappreciated by their husbands and for discordant wives to actually receive less in the way of nonverbal positives from their husbands (Noller, 1987). In addition, the spouses of depressed patients may be particularly critical of them, rather than affirming of them, even in the context of offering help (Hautzinger et al., 1982). Further, since low self-esteem may serve as a vulnerability factor for depression (Brown, Andrews, Harris, Adler, & Bridge, 1986), one might suspect that affirmation by the spouse, when effective, could reduce the probability of future episodes of depression and reinforce maintenance of gains made in therapy. Clearly, the perception that the spouse is critical can promote relapse of depression (Hooley & Teasdale, 1989). Someone who sees her husband as being appreciative, complimentary, and affirming, on the other hand, may well be better able to tolerate threats to self-esteem arising from stresses external to the relationship and remain symptom-free despite challenging circumstances.

## SPOUSAL DEPENDABILITY

A fifth aspect of social support can be labeled spousal dependability, or the perceived presence of a "reliable alliance" (Weiss, 1974), that is, the perception that supportive others *would be available* if they were needed. The perception that supportive others would be available if needed may directly increase perceived control over the environment (Glass & Singer, 1972), reducing reactivity to stressful situations. Confirming the importance of perceived reliable alliance, Lieberman (1982) found that persons perceiving their world as containing significant others (particularly spouses) who could be counted on were less likely to be affected by stress. At a minimum, the spouse who believes the partner can be counted on will perceive him/herself as having greater resources with which to face difficulties as they arise.

Of primary importance for the sense of spousal dependability is the perception that the partner is committed to the relationship and that separation or divorce is unlikely. Unfortunately, in the context of co-occurring marital discord and depression there is rarely a sense of spousal dependability, and, as might be expected, this often leads to a sense of great personal vulnerability (cf. Weiss, 1974). In addition, Beach and Tesser (1987) hypothesized that the perception that one's spouse is committed to the relationship should have a positive impact on trust and the willingness to engage in the self-disclosures characteristic of intimacy. Thus establishing a sense of spousal dependability and the perception that one's spouse is committed to the relationship may be an additional precursor to the emergence or reemergence of confiding and intimacy in the relationship.

INTIMACY AND CONFIDING

Finally, a sixth aspect of social support of relevance to mood is the possible direct induction of positive affect and the concurrent sense of well-being that can result from intimate exchanges with a spouse (cf. Beach & Tesser, 1987; Weiss, 1974). Intimacy in this context refers to a relationship in which innermost feelings, thoughts, and dispositions can be revealed and explored (cf. Waring, 1988). Intimacy is typically expected to increase and deepen as a relationship develops (Altman & Taylor, 1973). In addition, as would be expected, intimacy is associated with marital satisfaction (Fitzpatrick, 1987), and sustaining intimacy may predict higher levels of marital satisfaction at midlife (McAdams & Vaillant, 1982). Beach and Tesser (1987) proposed that intimacy involves taking a risk by engaging in behaviors that carry some uncertainty as to the spouse's evaluative response. This in turn should be expected to be related to strong arousal and potentially strong positive or negative emotion, depending on the spouse's acceptance or nonacceptance of the self-disclosure. Thus taking a risk by revealing something deeply personal to one's spouse when coupled with spousal acceptance should be a powerful mood elevator and engender strong feelings of attraction and love. Conversely, sharing of one's self when coupled with subsequent criticism or rejection can produce powerful dysphoria and anger (Green & Murray, 1973). In the context of marital discord, the loss of trust engendered by the ongoing discord should serve to powerfully inhibit self-disclosure. In addition, when a spouse does self-disclose, the probability of a rejecting response by the partner is likely to be higher in the context of maritally discordant than in a nondiscordant relationship. Given the depressed person's tendency to avoid negative outcomes and use passive coping strategies, one might anticipate that intimacy would be particularly vulnerable to deterioration in the context of co-occurring marital discord and depression.

A primary component of intimacy as it has been defined above is the act of confiding. The presence of a confiding relationship has been found to play a central role in vulnerability to depression (Brown & Harris, 1978; Brown & Prudo, 1981; Costello, 1982; Lin, Dean, & Ensel, 1986; Roy, 1978; Solomon & Bromet, 1982). While the exact mechanism by which confiding protects against depression is not fully understood, it is possible that, in addition to the direct production of positive affect as outlined above, it works to reduce the incidence of depression by providing increased opportunities for direct provision of aid and advice, increased opportunities for self-esteem support, and decreased avoidance of problem areas. As discussed earlier, having a confiding relationship probably presupposes having a partner who is available for cohesive activities, is perceived as being accepting of emotional expression, is seen as being dependable and committed, and is more likely to be affirming than rejecting. In sum, confiding may be a marker for or instrumental in producing each of the prominent sources of support in the marital relationship. It is not surprising, then, that it has been related so robustly to depressive symptomatology.

## CONCLUSIONS

Unfortunately, in the presence of marital distress, the six forms of social support outlined above may appear inaccessible. Indeed, marital distress is often associated with loss of feelings of trust, closeness, and love for the spouse (O'Leary, Fincham, & Turkewitz, 1983), making the spouse seem less available as an attractive source of cohesive interaction, less available as someone who will listen to problems, less available to give helpful advice, less likely to provide support to one's self-esteem, less likely to appear dependable and committed, and less likely to be a target of intimate exchanges. Because of their importance for depressive symptoms, it is these aspects of social support in the context of marriage that we will address most directly in our recommendations for treatment.

## Marital Discord and the Production of Stress

As research on stress has proliferated, a variety of perspectives have emerged. However, from the standpoint of guiding therapeutic intervention, we have found it useful to confine ourselves to the identification of highly probable, concrete marital stressors; that is, we have been interested in finding those events or conditions within the marital relationship that are most strongly and consistently related to felt stress and depressive symptomatology. Life event research helps by highlighting the dimensions that tend to exacerbate felt stress or depressive symptomatology. For example, it is now clear that it is the quality of life events—that is, their positive or negative nature rather than simply the amount of change entailed in adjusting to them—that is most related to depression (Brown & Harris, 1986). Likewise, it is chronic, or repetitious, stressors that carry the greatest potential for producing strong stress responses (Pearlin & Lieberman, 1979). In addition, stressors are most likely to produce a strong stress response and depression if they carry the possibility of threat or danger (cf. Brown & Harris, 1978; Mandler, 1982).

Importantly, depressed patients report feeling more vulnerable to marriage- and family-related stresses than to other stressors (Schless, Schwartz, Goetz, & Mendels, 1974).

Following the stress literature, we have found it useful to identify only those high-intensity, negative, threatening, and recurrent patterns as marital stressors requiring direct attention. This distinction is useful clinically, because when high-intensity stressors of the type discussed below can be identified, they often need to be given priority in treatment. When not addressed, they appear to block recovery for the patient. However, it is the individual's perception or appraisal of the event that is critical in determining the magnitude of the stress response (Lazarus & Folkman, 1986). Accordingly, there is often considerable value in therapeutic intervention aimed at changing perceptions of behavior or attributions of spousal behavior as well as changing dysfunctional interaction patterns. Likewise, idiosyncratic patterns that may be perceived as intensely stressful by a given couple or individual cannot be ignored simply because they do not fit into the categories outlined below.

Several patterns of marital behavior that occur rather commonly in discordant, depressed couples are negative, chronic, and pregnant with threat. In particular, we have found it clinically useful to address (1) verbal and physical aggression, (2) threats of separation and divorce, (3) severe spousal denigration, criticism, and blame, and (4) severe disruption of scripted routines. Of course, major stressors that are idiosyncratic to a couple are also addressed.


## VERBAL AND PHYSICAL AGGRESSION

It is quite well documented that discordant, depressed couples show considerable hostility and tension in their interactions (Kahn et al., 1985). Clinically we have seen couples in which long periods of felt isolation and relative silence were punctuated by outbursts of accusation and recrimination. Even more destructive is a pattern we have observed involving rapidly escalating arguments culminating in violence. Interactional patterns of this type leave even nondepressed spouses exhausted and drained. For depressed spouses, they provide a level of stress well beyond the level that allows for symptomatic recovery. For recovered individuals, this pattern may be expected to lead to relapse into depression. Indeed, Paykel and colleagues (1969) found that the most frequent event preceding the *onset* of depression was an increase in marital arguments. Thus, when we see a pattern of high-intensity arguments associated with physical or verbal abuse, this becomes a very early target of treatment.

## THREATS OF SEPARATION AND DIVORCE

A less discussed stressor associated with marital discord is the fear of marital separation and divorce. Depressed, discordant couples are often plagued by a sense of uncertainty about the future of their relationship. A frequent concern of couples entering therapy is that if the problems they are experiencing are not quickly resolved, marital separation may be imminent. Marital separation and divorce have been documented as major stressors in their own right (Bloom, Asher, & White, 1978). However, the role of fear of separation in the production of stress has been less well investigated. With a 49% divorce rate (Glick, 1984) projected for first marriages formed in the 1980s, however, concern about divorce could represent a significant element linking marital discord to stress. This uncertainty about the future of the relationship can often be conceptualized as a low level of perceived reliable alliance, to be dealt with in due course during marital therapy, particularly when doubts about the viability of the marriage are only moderate and largely unspoken. However, we have also seen spouses trade the threat of divorce as a potent way of underscoring a point during disagreements. It is this pattern that we view as falling into the more malignant marital stressor category. For the depressed spouse, there is often some appeal to the idea of divorce, since it can come to represent escape and surcease. For the nondepressed spouse, the threat of divorce may be presented as a realistic representation of the level of frustration felt with the depressed partner. Divorce represents an opportunity to create needed distance from the spouse, and the use of the threat of divorce is often rewarded by some increased distance. Thus explicit spoken statements about divorce or actions that strongly imply thoughts of divorce can become established aspects of a couple's ongoing interaction in the context of discord and depression. In our clinical experience such events are not uncommon and can be very disruptive to therapy if not addressed promptly. Accordingly, when this pattern is observed, it constitutes a direct target for intervention very early in therapy.

## SEVERE SPOUSAL DENIGRATION, CRITICISM, AND BLAME

As discussed above, it is clear that feedback from the spouse plays an important role in self-evaluation. Thus the chronic use of statements that denigrate or devalue the partner should take a considerable toll on self-esteem over time. In addition, spousal criticism appears to be related to more maladaptive coping and less adaptive coping, contributing to further decrements in adjustment over time (Manne & Zautra, 1989). In the context of depression and marital discord, devaluation of the partner can go from being nonverbal and implicit to being directly stated in harsh and uncompromising terms. Some spouses may explosively make vulgar references to their depressed partners or call them lazy, worthless, and bad. Others may criticize and treat their depressed partners as inferiors. At low levels this type of behavior may be seen as providing neither self-esteem support nor affirmation. As such, it is dealt with in an ongoing way throughout therapy. However, when a shift occurs from low-level stress to the high-level stress caused by explicit denunciation, devaluation represents a major stressor, a threat to remission of depressive symptoms, and a likely source of relapse. As such, it must be dealt with explicitly and very early in marital therapy for depression.

## SEVERE DISRUPTION OF SCRIPTED ROUTINES

A fourth common source of stress in discordant, depressed marriages arises from the breakdown of cohesion and the resulting disruption of routine scripted marital behavior (e.g., no kiss good-bye in the morning, a breakdown of the usual division of accepted responsibilities, non-responsiveness to partner-initiated interaction). When a script is disrupted, the individual is forced to search for new ways to cope with the situation. This is likely to lead to increasingly erratic and random coping attempts, which increases the likelihood of sustained emotional arousal, exhaustion, and illness. In the presence of preexisting low self-esteem, this process appears likely to be intensified (Taylor & Brown, 1988). As Lewinsohn and colleagues (1985) pointed out, disruption of scripts also produces increased self-awareness, the symptoms of which include self-criticism (Duval & Wicklund, 1972), negative expectancies (Carver, Blaney, & Scheier, 1979), and intensification of mood-induction procedures (Scheier & Carver, 1977). It is possible to view marital discord as typically involving two spouses who are doing their best to disrupt each other's scripted, automatic behavior. To the extent that this behavior is low level, it can be conceptualized as reflecting a low level of couple cohesion. Disruption of scripted behavior can occur from such low-level events as increased hesitancy in interaction and reluctance to communicate. In such cases, the disruption is likely to be adequately resolved by interventions aimed at building new forms of marital support and cohesion. However, when the disruption introduced is severe, such as the disruption that can be produced by threatening to move out of the house, routinely missing the family dinner hour, routinely staying late at work to minimize contact with the spouse, or refusing all physical contact with the spouse, it may set into motion very powerful depressogenic processes

(Oatley & Bolton, 1985). In such cases, the disruption of major routines may need to be addressed before any progress is likely to be forthcoming in the relief of depressive symptoms. In particular, it may be necessary to help couples reestablish routines from some earlier point in their relationship.


CONCLUSIONS

Identifying major stressors in the marriage early in therapy and reducing them is critical if a positive focus is to emerge in the early phase of therapy. Accordingly, careful assessment for the common major stressors outlined above, as well as for major stressors idiosyncratic to the couple, should have high priority in the initial sessions of therapy.


## Depression in the Production and Maintenance of Marital Discord

It appears that the long-term presence of depressive symptoms may produce a further exacerbation of marital discord (Beach, Arias, & O'Leary, 1989). The depressed person is likely to have a negative impact on others (Biglan et al., 1989), and this might be expected to intensify the negative feelings experienced by his/her partner. Depressed, discordant couples often establish a strong pattern of avoidance and "suffering in silence," with occasional angry outbursts punctuating the tension. This pattern is unlikely to be effective in resolving marital issues as they arise, leading to an increasing backlog of unsettled problems over time. Spouses of depressed persons who are in distressed marriages are also likely to experience their partners' depressive behavior as manipulative and accusatory (Bullock, Siegel, Weissman, & Paykel, 1972). They are still angry—or even more angry—after the display of depressive behavior but are likely to feel that they can say nothing. As such, the depressive behavior is likely to add to the resentments that already exist, while derailing the nondepressed spouse's attempts to raise conflictual issues for discussion. As the duration of the depression and marital discord increases, the amount of rejection by the nondepressed spouse is likely to increase (Nelson & Beach, in press; Winer, Bonner, Blaney, & Murray, 1981) and the marital relationship is likely to continue to deteriorate.

Depression has also been associated with a variety of behavioral deficits that might be expected to further aggravate ongoing marital distress. The depressed spouse is likely to make less eye contact (Hinch-liffe, Lancashire, & Roberts, 1970) with the nondepressed spouse, make fewer comments that facilitate problem solving (Biglan et al., 1985), be slower in making responses (Libet & Lewinsohn, 1973), and be a poorer problem solver (Gotlib & Asarnow, 1979). In addition, common symptoms of depression include avoidance of others, difficulty concentrating on a topic, and loss of interest in previously gratifying behavior. While these consequences of depression might be expected to put a strain on even the best relationships, they clearly limit the capacity of the dyad containing a depressed member to make progress in resolving preexisting marital distress without the help of a third party.

The characteristic coping styles of depressed individuals may also tend to limit their ability to reverse the course of marital discord once it is initiated. As discussed earlier, depressed individuals appear prone to use high levels of both confrontation and escape, and to feel both angry and fearful (Folkman & Lazarus, 1986). Accordingly, they are likely to vacillate in a self-defeating manner when confronted with interpersonal situations that should be handled by confident and decisive action (Kessler et al., 1985), leading to brief hostile exchanges followed by withdrawal. In addition, as the depressed individual becomes more focused on him/herself and his/her own flaws (cf. Pyszczynski & Greenberg, 1987), this focus away from direct confrontation of difficulties and problems would be expected to be particularly ineffective in dealing with marital discord (cf. Pearlin & Schooler, 1978). Thus it seems likely that as the relationship between marital discord and depression unfolds, an increasingly vicious cycle is established.

This vicious cycle may feed on itself until it is eventually terminated by either divorce, suicide, or successful amelioration of the difficulties through outside intervention or change in circumstances. It appears that divorce may be one common resolution of this vicious cycle. Merikangas (1984) found a dramatically increased rate of divorce in depressed patients 2 years after discharge from a psychiatric facility, reporting a rate nine times that of the general population. Beach, Winters, and Weintraub (1986) also reported a sharply elevated rate of divorce following discharge from the hospital for depressed patients. Similarly, suicide may be a common resolution of the vicious cycle represented by depression and marital discord. Suicide is elevated in the recently divorced and separated, and ongoing marital discord appears to be associated with higher than normal rates of suicidal ideation and behavior (Schneidman, Farberow, & Litman, 1979; Slater & Depue, 1981). Indeed, feelings of isolation from those considered closest and little affection shown by the marital partner emerged as the factors best differentiating the suicide attempters from community controls in a recent study (Welz, 1988). Thus marital discord and depression may tend to be mutually maintaining when untreated and lead jointly to particularly poor prognosis.

On a more positive note, however, it has recently been found that in a structured situation where disclosure of interpersonal problems with the other is expected and encouraged, disclosure between depressed persons and others can be positive and productive. Indeed, it appears to "clear the air" and improve mood in both participants in the interaction (Burchill & Stiles, 1988). It appears, then, that the negative mood induction posited by Coyne (1976) and found by Biglan and colleagues (1989) may occur only in the context of avoidance and frustration, not when self-disclosure and direct problem solving are supported and expected. Thus intervention is probably necessary to break the cycle of chronic marital discord and recurring depression in an optimal manner, but there is good reason to believe that structured intervention can reverse the vicious cycle represented by marital discord and depression.

## The Role of Cognition

As has been alluded to above, we certainly do believe there is a role for cognition in understanding the interrelationships between depressive symptomatology and marital discord. We have used terms such as perceived support, self-focus, and script disruption in describing the relationships already addressed. It is obvious these constructs could be best elaborated within a cognitive framework. It is important to note, however, that marital discord is the clear focus of the model being developed and we believe the marital relationship provides a very promising focus for intervention at each of the points elaborated above. We welcome the opportunity to blend newer cognitive marital techniques (cf. Baucom & Epstein, 1990; Epstein, Schlesinger, & Dryden, 1988) with the approaches which we have used successfully with a depressive and discordant population. Indeed, behavioral marital therapy has had many "cognitive" elements from its beginning. We envision the incorporation of specifically marital cognitive interventions as they are shown to increase the effectiveness of marital therapy in general, or increase the response of depressed and maritally discordant patients in particular to marital therapy (cf. Beach & Bauserman, 1990). In addition, there may be times when a blending of individual cognitive therapy (Beck et al., 1979) or individual interpersonal therapy (Klerman et al., 1984) with marital therapy may be the most reasonable approach (cf. Dobson, Jacobson, & Victor, 1988).

## The Case of Severe Pathology

For the most part, the model we are proposing (see Figure 3-2) is meant to highlight the role of marital variables in the production of depressive symptoms. We believe, however, that multiple causal elements are often at work when an individual succumbs to an episode of depression. It is not unusual for persons presenting for treatment to give evidence of a history of social reticence, chronic low self-esteem, and perhaps a family history of affective disorder. The models reviewed in Chapter 2 often highlight points of therapeutic intervention that fall at least partially outside the domain of the marriage and that may be important to address in order to facilitate a given individual's recovery. In the case of very severe depression that possibly requires hospitalization, the evidence suggests that a significant genetic diathesis for affective disorder may be present. In contrast to mild to moderately depressed individuals, the more severely depressed also appear to respond poorly to nonspecific supportive interventions combined with placebo and show an enhanced response to active antidepressant medication (Elkin et al., 1989). This suggests that for more severely depressed patients, interventions targeted directly at the individual's symptoms of depression (i.e., cognitive, interpersonal, or pharmacological intervention) may be an appropriate preliminary step prior to beginning marital therapy. Clinically, we have seen cases of depression in which the patient was sufficiently depressed that completing marital assignments was unlikely; in such cases, an unhealthy therapeutic focus on the depressed individual rather than the relationship seemed all too likely. In cases of severe depression, then, marital intervention may need to be delayed until the patient's depression is at least somewhat improved. Improving the depression through individual or somatic approaches should decrease avoidance of marital issues and enhance the chances that marital therapy will work. However, the marital discord model predicts that in the presence of unremitting marital discord, somatic or individual interventions are likely to be followed by incomplete recovery, early relapse, or divorce (cf. Hooley & Teasdale, 1989; Tennant, Bebbington, & Hurry, 1981; Paykel & Tanner, 1976). Thus marital discord should be assessed, and where present, addressed, in all depressed populations.

The marital model of depression that emerges from the above considerations is portrayed in Figure 3-2. This extended marital model highlights the importance of six distinct areas of support within the marital dyad as well as the role of the dyad in carrying major stressors. Both stressors and supports are hypothesized to have direct effects on depression. While not shown in the schematic representation of the

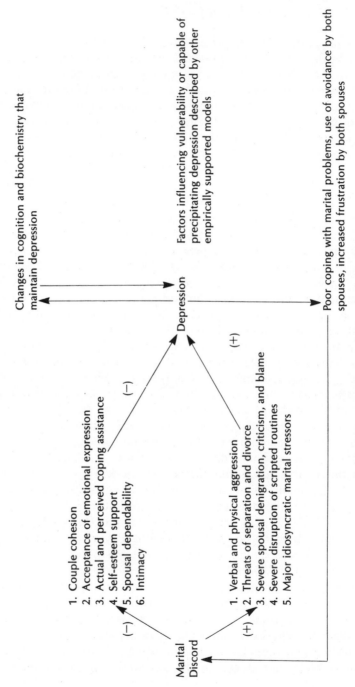

**FIGURE 3-2.** An elaborated marital discord model of depression.

model, it is also hypothesized that support within the dyad helps to buffer stressors arising external to the relationship. Finally, depressive symptomatology is shown to be influenced by factors arising outside the marital context and more amenable to analysis from other perspectives. Once established, depressive symptomatology is hypothesized to exacerbate marital discord in a number of ways and to produce a strong tendency in both spouses to avoid dealing with marital problems. This in turn is hypothesized to contribute to a vicious cycle of decreasing marital adjustment and increasing depression.

## Translating Theory into Action

A sensitive issue for the field of psychotherapy is how one uses the systematic observations of researchers to inform and guide the psychotherapy process. Clearly, there is more of a gap between clinical research and practice than is desirable (Barlow, 1980). When practical intervention is attempted in the absence of relevant information, the result is likely to be less than optimal therapy. This reflects negatively on the field of psychotherapy as a whole. Conversely, when researchers sift through the relevant data to produce a highly specified treatment approach, it is often clear to therapists that the approach is little better (or even worse) than the idiosyncratic, intuitive approach it was meant to replace. This occurs when therapeutic approaches are presented in an overly "packaged" manner that renders them inadequate for application to real patients who have a multiplicity of idiosyncrasies and special concerns. Applying packaged treatment approaches as they are commonly presented often seems rather like trying to fit everyone into a size nine shoe; most people are going to end up being at least a little uncomfortable.

The approach we recommend with regard to depression is one that recognizes the multiple causal models that can be appropriately applied to the formation and maintenance of depressive symptomatology. When marital discord is present, then the marital discord model should be used to help identify important points of intervention. Other models may also be useful in illuminating the needs of a particular patient. But in each case, the points of intervention are best defined by empirically supported models. At each point of therapeutuic intervention there may be a large number of techniques that could produce equivalent therapeutic effects. In the material that follows, we present a variety of techniques from the marital therapy literature that address the different points of intervention highlighted in the marital discord model of depression. As powerful new techniques are developed, borrowed from other theoretical orientations, or suggested by more basic experimental work, they can be readily added to this approach. Indeed, the great advantage of the models approach is that it stimulates clinical creativity while maintaining a solid grounding in the relevant research literature. In the upcoming chapters we will share the techniques we have used to date and provide information of importance for successfully conducting marital therapy with depressed individuals.

# II

## TREATMENT OF CO-OCCURRING DEPRESSION AND MARITAL DISCORD

# 4

## Overview of Therapy: Assessment, Process, and the Therapist's Role in Marital Therapy for Depression

This chapter provides an overview of marital therapy for depression. First, we focus on assessment issues. In particular, we highlight the areas of psychopathology and marital process that require assessment if an informed decision regarding the most appropriate form of intervention for a depressed, discordant couple is to be forthcoming. Next we highlight several process issues and discuss strategies for staying on track through a variety of potentially difficult therapy situations. We then discuss the therapist's many roles in conducting marital therapy for depression. Finally, we provide a brief session-by-session outline of therapy. It is hoped that this chapter will help therapists match their treatment to the couple more effectively, remain alert to the subtle nuances of therapy that can be consequential as the process unfolds, and more effectively guide the couple to a successful outcome.

### What Is Marital Therapy for Depression?

Marital therapy for depression is typically relatively brief and focused on changing ongoing problem behavior. As can be seen in Figure 4-1, the therapist using marital therapy for depression will apply a series of interventions in three phases. First, the therapist will focus on identifying

| STAGE I | STAGE II | STAGE III |
|---|---|---|
| Rapidly eliminate major stressors and enhance couple cohesion, caring, and companionship | Restructure communication and interaction to build stable, functional relationship | Enhance maintenance, focus on relapse prevention |

$\longrightarrow$ between Stage I and Stage II, $\longrightarrow$ between Stage II and Stage III

FIGURE 4-1. The flow of therapy.

and rapidly eliminating extreme stressors within the relationship and reestablishing joint positive activities within the relationship. When successfully implemented, this stage of therapy will often produce a substantial elevation in mood for the depressed patient and increased expressions of positive feelings on the part of both spouses. This initial boost in morale and positive feelings allows the couple to confront the second phase of therapy, which involves the restructuring of the marital relationship.

The second phase of therapy is focused on the way the spouses communicate, solve problems, and interact on a day-to-day basis. This phase of therapy provides the couple with a more supportive pattern of problem resolution; it systematically increases the support value of the relationship in the areas of acceptance of emotional expression, actual and perceived coping assistance, perceived spousal dependability, and couple intimacy. During this phase of therapy, there will typically be further decreases in the stress previously associated with coercive patterns of exchange within the dyad. Relationship cohesion and self-esteem support are likely to receive some additional attention during this phase of therapy, but they will typically be less a focus of attention than during the first phase of therapy. When successfully implemented, this phase of therapy leaves the couple better integrated and better able to handle difficulties they may encounter in the future.

The third phase of therapy has as its focus preparing the couple for termination, requiring the therapist to take a less directive stance. In this final phase of therapy, the therapist is interested primarily in helping the client couple identify likely high-risk situations that may produce either relapse of depressive symptoms or return of marital discord. Vulnerabilities for further problems and warning signs are reviewed. The therapist prepares the couple to expect, and be accepting of, transitory symptoms of both depression and marital discord. Appropriate ways of coping with a return of depressive symptoms or marital discord are reviewed. During this final phase, the therapist helps the couple attribute their gains in therapy to their caring and love for each other.

## When Is Marital Therapy for Depression Appropriate for a Couple?

As alluded to in Chapter 3, we do not believe that every discordant couple with a depressed member is likely to show appreciable benefit from marital intervention. Accordingly, the therapist must decide if marital therapy makes sense for *this* couple given *these* circumstances, *this* symptom picture, and the state of their marital relationship at *this* point in time. We believe marital therapy as a primary or solitary intervention modality is appropriate when the following considerations have been satisfied: (1) the risk of suicide has been carefully assessed and risk of precipitous suicidal gestures has been determined to be low; (2) the depressed patient has received a thorough diagnostic assessment and has been accurately diagnosed as nonbipolar (i.e., receives a diagnosis of either major depression, unipolar type, or dysthymia), and neither psychotic features nor organic mood disorders are present; (3) the presence of marital discord has been clearly established; (4) marital discord appears to play an etiological or maintaining role in the depression; (5) both spouses have been seen individually and assessed for hidden agendas, desire for immediate divorce, low level of commitment to work on improving the marriage, and presence of extramarital sexual activity, and the therapist has some confidence that both spouses are interested in working at improving their marital relationship. If these conditions are not met, it is likely that marital therapy should be used later, or in conjunction with other treatments, or perhaps not at all. We consider each assessment issue in turn below.

## Assessment of Psychopathology

### HIGH SUICIDAL POTENTIAL

The most obvious complication for marital therapists working with depressed patients is suicidal ideation and suicidal intent. It is, of course, necessary to assess for suicidal potential with every depressed patient. It should not be assumed that simply because a patient does not voice suicidal feelings or plans that no suicidal ideation is present. It is important to explore with every patient any thoughts they may have had about harming themselves, either actively or passively. This will typically be best accomplished during an initial individual assessment session. Depression occurring in the context of poor marital support is associated with a particular proneness to suicidal ideation and behavior (Slater &

Depue, 1981; Thomssen & Möller, 1988; Welz, Veiel, & Hafner, 1988).
Thus the marital therapist dealing with depressed patients must always be
particularly concerned with these issues.

When suicidal ideation is acknowledged by the depressed patient, a
full exploration of the ideation and its associated features should follow.
The strength of the wish to live and current reasons for living should be
assessed, as should the strength of the wish to die. The duration, frequency, and perceived control over suicidal urges need to be explored
carefully, as does the extent to which the patient may actively reject the
thoughts and urges when they occur. Finally, the nature of any plan, its
degree of elaboration, its feasibility, and the patient's readiness to act on
the plan formulated should be assessed. In our own clinical work we
follow the guidelines offered by Beck's Scale for Suicide Ideation (Table
4-1). This scale provides a compact format for assessing the relative
lethality of suicidal ideation.

When suicidal ideation is weak, transitory, and felt to be under the
patient's control, and when no plan is being actively pursued, suicidal
ideation may be accepted by the therapist as one of the "normal" manifestations of depression. While the depressed patient should be told to
keep the therapist informed of any increase in suicidal ideation, there is
little reason to see low levels of suicidal ideation as being a contraindication for marital therapy. Conversely, when suicidal ideation is strong,
persistent, and compelling, and when plans are being considered and
elaborated, the therapist must be more concerned. While the current
evidence suggests that available social support and a confiding relationship are particularly important in such cases (Thomssen & Möller, 1988)
and may contribute to the difference between mild and severe suicidal
intent, we have found it difficult to maintain a consistent dyadic focus
with suicidal patients, and marital therapy has been compromised as a
result.

In our own pilot work comparing marital therapy for depression and
cognitive therapy for depression with a suicidal population (O'Leary,
Sandeen, & Beach, 1987), we found a more reliable effect on level of
depression using cognitive therapy. We suspect the "failure" of marital
therapy in these cases has to do with the difficulty the therapist and the
couple experience in focusing on marital issues when strong suicidal
ideation is present. Thus it seems most reasonable with patients displaying high levels of severe suicidal ideation to propose a somewhat longer
course of therapy, one that begins with individual work and proceeds to
marital work as they are more able to benefit from a dyadic focus.

When suicidal ideation is weak or absent, or suicide potential is
judged to be relatively low, suicide typically will not remain a topic of
continuing intensive assessment. The Beck Depression Inventory (BDI),

TABLE 4-1. Scale for Suicide Ideation (for Ideators)

Name _____ Date _____

Day of                                                Time of crisis/most
interview                                             severe point of illness

I. *Characteristics of attitude toward living/dying*

( )   1. Wish to live                                                    ( )
         0. Moderate to strong
         1. Weak
         2. None
( )   2. Wish to die                                                     ( )
         0. None
         1. Weak
         2. Moderate to strong
( )   3. Reasons for living/dying                                        ( )
         0. For living outweigh for dying
         1. About equal
         2. For dying outweigh for living
( )   4. Desire to make active suicide attempt                          ( )
         0. None
         1. Weak
         2. Moderate to strong
( )   5. Passive suicidal attempt                                        ( )
         0. Would take precautions to save life
         1. Would leave life/death to chance (e.g., carelessly cross-
            ing a busy street)
         2. Would avoid steps necessary to save or maintain life
            (e.g., diabetic ceasing to take insulin)

If all four code entries for items 4 and 5 are "0," skip sections II, III, and IV, and enter "8"—
"not applicable"—in each of the blank code spaces.

II. *Characteristics of suicide ideation/wish*

( )   6. Time dimension duration                                        ( )
         0. Brief, fleeting periods
         1. Longer periods
         2. Continuous (chronic), or almost continuous
( )   7. Time dimension: frequency                                      ( )
         0. Rare, occasional
         1. Intermittent
         2. Persistent or continuous
( )   8. Attitude toward ideation/wish                                  ( )
         0. Rejecting
         1. Ambivalent; indifferent
         2. Accepting

*(continued)*

TABLE 4-1. (Continued)

( )  9. Control over suicidal action/acting-out wish                    ( )
        0. Has sense of control
        1. Unsure of control
        2. Has no sense of control
( ) 10. Deterrents to active attempt (e.g., family, religion; serious    ( )
        injury if unsuccessful; irreversible)
        0. Would not suicide because of a deterrent
        1. Some concern about deterrents
        2. Minimal or no concern about deterrents
        (Indicate deterrents, if any): _____

( ) 11. Reason for contemplated attempt                                  ( )
        0. To manipulate the environment, get attention, revenge
        1. Combination of "0" and "2"
        2. Escape, surcease, solve problems

### III. *Characteristics of contemplated attempts*

( ) 12. Method: specificity/planning                                     ( )
        0. Not considered
        1. Considered, but details not worked out
        2. Details worked out/well formulated
( ) 13. Method: availability/opportunity                                 ( )
        0. Method not available; no opportunity
        1. Method would take time/effort; opportunity not really
           available
        2a. Method and opportunity available
        2b. Future opportunity or availability of method
            anticipated
( ) 14. Sense of "capability" to carry out attempt                       ( )
        0. No courage, too weak, afraid, incompetent
        1. Unsure of courage, competence
        2. Sure of competence, courage
( ) 15. LEAVE BLANK                                                      ( )
( ) 16. Expectancy/anticipation of actual attempt                        ( )
        0. No
        1. Uncertain, not sure
        2. Yes
( ) 17. LEAVE BLANK                                                      ( )

### IV. *Actualization of contemplated attempt*

( ) 18. Actual preparation                                               ( )
        0. None
        1. Partial (e.g., starting to collect pills)
        2. Complete (e.g., had pills, razor, loaded gun)
( ) 19. Suicide note                                                     ( )
        0. None
        1. Started but not completed or deposited; only thought
           about
        2. Completed; deposited

*(continued)*

TABLE 4-1. (Continued)

---

( )  20. Final acts in anticipation of death (insurance, will, gifts,                    ( )
         etc.)
         0. None
         1. Thought about or made some arrangements
         2. Made definite plans or completed arrangements
( )  21. Deception/concealment of contemplated attempt                                   ( )
         0. Revealed ideas openly
         1. Held back on revealing
         2. Attempted to deceive, conceal, lie

V. *Background factors*

( )  22. Previous suicide attempts                                                       ( )
         0. None
         1. One
         2. More than one
( )  23. Intent to die associated with last attempt                                      ( )
         (if N/A enter "8")
         0. Low
         1. Moderate; ambivalent, unsure
         2. High

---

completed regularly over the course of therapy, can provide a brief, convenient, ongoing assessment of suicidal ideation in such cases. The BDI can be self-administered by most depressed persons in about 5–10 minutes. The item assessing suicidal ideation asks the patient to choose the response that best reflects the way he/she is feeling. The options range from "I don't have any thoughts of killing myself" to "I would kill myself if I had the chance." The use of the BDI also allows the therapist to monitor the overall severity of the depression on an ongoing basis. The most generally used guidelines for determining level of severity from the BDI are: (1) a BDI score of less than 10 indicates no or minimal depression, (2) a BDI score between 10 and 18 indicates mild to moderate depression, (3) a BDI score between 19 and 29 indicates moderate to severe depression, and (4) a BDI score between 30 and 63 indicates severe depression (Beck, Steer, & Garbin, 1988). Because of its ease and utility, we strongly recommend use of the BDI routinely throughout therapy. The BDI may be ordered from the Psychological Corporation, Order Service Center, P.O. Box 839954, San Antonio, TX 78283-9954.

PRESENCE OF ACTIVE PSYCHOSIS

In our own outpatient work we have not been faced frequently with patients who had mood congruent or mood incongruent psychotic features as part of their presenting problems. However, this constellation of problems is not uncommon in inpatient settings. Clinicians in hospital settings attempting to apply the marital discord model of depression are more likely to encounter patients who have mood congruent or mood incongruent psychotic features. It is our impression that such patients are not good candidates for marital therapy during their actively psychotic phase (cf. Clarkin, Haas, & Glick, 1988). However, as their psychotic features clear and as they become somewhat less depressed, marital therapy may begin to be an attractive adjunct to somatic and individual therapies. Therapists doing marital therapy in inpatient settings, however, are likely to need a heavier emphasis on educating the spouse who is not affectively ill about depression (cf. Clarkin et al., 1988; Falloon, Hole, Mulroy, Norris, & Pembleton, 1988). With appropriate changes, it is likely that a focus on reducing ongoing marital discord will be helpful both in elevating mood and building a foundation for prevention of relapse (Hooley, Orley, & Teasdale, 1986; Hooley & Teasdale, 1989). In addition, it may be possible to avoid the extremely high rates of divorce that typically follow hospitalization for depressive episodes (Merikangas et al., 1979; Beach et al., 1986).

DIAGNOSIS OF BIPOLAR DISORDER

We believe marital therapy is appropriate for bipolar patients who are maritally discordant, particularly if they are not currently in a depressed or manic episode. However, current evidence suggests that many bipolar patients will require pharmacological intervention either prophylactically or in response to episodic symptoms as their primary treatment modality. To the extent that stress and support are shown to play a role in the triggering of initial bipolar episodes or relapses (e.g., Miklowitz, Goldstein, Nuechterlein, Snyder, & Doane, 1986), addressing family and marital discord may be helpful in lessening the frequency of relapse of bipolar disorder, or perhaps reducing the risk of onset in high-risk individuals. Skills in problem-solving discussion as well as listening skills, both engendered in marital therapy, may be helpful in gaining the patient's compliance with appropriate somatic treatments. This issue, however, requires additional study. Thus it may be that marital and family therapies can improve the outcome of standard somatic interventions for bipolar disorder (Clarkin et al., 1988). Importantly, however, bipolar patients in a depressive episode should not be considered equivalent to unipolar depressed patients. Accordingly, careful assessment of the patient's history of psychopathology and accurate diagnosis are important preliminary steps in applying the marital discord model to depressed, discordant couples.

## DIAGNOSIS OF ORGANIC MOOD DISORDER

Marital therapy will not be sufficient to alleviate entirely depressive symptomatology that is secondary to organic factors. For example, if a patient with thyroid disease or neoplasm initially presents as depressed, there is no good reason to expect that marital therapy, even if successful in building a stronger relationship, will alleviate entirely the depressed mood or feelings of fatigue. While such individuals may present rather infrequently for outpatient psychotherapy, therapists should nonetheless be aware of the possibility that physical illness may, at times, be confused with depression. Helpful guides for mental health workers who may need to be alert to signs of physical impairment or disease are available (e.g., Berg et al., 1987; Hales 1986). Should any organic factors be suspected, referral for appropriate laboratory work should be done expeditiously. Accordingly, a good working relationship with a physician is likely to be important to facilitate appropriate diagnosis and treatment.

## SEVERE PERSONALITY DISORDER

A significant percentage of persons presenting with marital discord and depression will show some evidence of preexisting personality disorder. In general, this is not of great significance with regard to the process of therapy. Mild personality disorder may slow down progress in therapy or make particular assignments more difficult, but it need not be a contraindication for marital therapy for depression. In particular, the relatively common situation of a depressed wife's also meeting criteria for mixed personality disorder with histrionic and dependent features requires little change in the standard course of therapy. In addition, apparent mild personality disorder will often resolve as symptomatic improvement in the depression occurs. However, if personality disorder becomes more severe, it can take on special significance and may require notable modification of the procedures outlined in this book. When a severe personality disorder appears to block the effective implementation of an even-handed dyadic focus, this should be considered a contraindication for marital work. The obstacle may be a short-term one, as when a temporary crisis is exacerbating the personality disorder, or may be more a long-standing one, as when an antisocial spouse is simply unavailable for or actively avoids productive marital work. While we do not recommend giving up on marital therapy for depression when an initial assessment indicates a high probability of severe personality disorder, it is prudent in such cases to predict a somewhat longer course of therapy and leave open the strong possibility that individual sessions will be used as necessary.

In our own clinical work, we have found it helpful at times to have spouses complete a Millon Clinical Multiaxial Inventory (Millon, 1983) to get a better sense of their personality styles. Alternatively, there are interview schedules of personality disorder that are keyed to the DSM-III-R diagnostic system (e.g., SCID-II; Spitzer, Williams, & Gibbon, 1987), and these can also provide guidance in the assessment of personality disorder in one or both spouses.

## Assessment of Marital Discord

### ONLY VERY MILD MARITAL DISCORD

In addition to conducting a careful assessment of the psychopathology being displayed by spouses, it is important to assess the marital environment being presented by the couple. Couples with more serious marital disturbances are likely to show poorer response to individual and somatic approaches (Vaughn & Leff, 1976), particularly if these problems do not improve over the course of therapy (Rounsaville et al., 1979a). Conversely, there is no available evidence that couples with a depressed spouse and only very mild marital discord will benefit from marital therapy for depression. We have used the Dyadic Adjustment Scale (DAS; Spanier, 1976; Table 4-2) as a measure of marital adjustment at the beginning of therapy. While its subscales have been questioned as distinct factors (Kazak, Jarmas, & Snitzer, 1988; Sharpley & Cross, 1982), the DAS remains a very useful instrument for indexing the level of discord in a relationship, and particular items and subscales can be clinically interesting. Accordingly, we recommend that clinicians use the DAS as the best available, brief assessment of the severity of marital discord. Recently, Jacobson (1989, personal communication) has suggested that both spouses obtaining a DAS score of 100 or less may predict a better response to marital therapy for depression. Our own clinical experience indicates the importance of the depressed wife's being clearly maritally discordant (i.e., DAS of 100 or less) but suggests that wives will often score somewhat lower on the DAS than their husbands. Thus couples with husbands scoring below the mean (115) on the DAS but above 100 may sometimes be appropriate for marital therapy for depression if their wives are scoring below 100.

Also useful clinically are more focused questionnaires such as the Areas of Change Questionnaire (ACQ; Margolin, Talovic, & Weinstein, 1983), the Feelings Questionnaire (FQ; O'Leary et al., 1983), the Marital Status Inventory (MSI; Weiss & Cerreto, 1980), the Marital Attributional Style Questionnaire (MASQ; Fincham, 1985), and the Broderick Commitment Scale (BCS; Beach & Broderick, 1983). Each of these measures assesses a potentially relevant dimension of the marital relationship. However, despite attempts to pull together a state-of-the-art package of marital measures (O'Leary, 1987), one of the "crucial challenges facing the marital therapy field in the '90's" is development of better measures of marital quality and interaction (Weiss & Heyman, 1990). Thus for the present a mainstay of marital assessment remains the marital interview, with self-report measures and informal observation of couple interactions supplementing the interview.

In the interview, therapists using the marital discord model of depression for guidance will carefully examine the areas of couple cohesion, acceptance of emotional expression, actual and perceived coping assistance, self-esteem support, perceived spousal dependability, and intimacy. Also receiving considerable direct assessment will be the stressor areas of overt hostility, threats of separation and divorce, severe spousal denigration, severe disruption of marital scripts, and major idosyncratic marital stressors. Within each category, the therapist will attempt to assess both the current level of the couple's functioning and the obstacles to change in a positive direction.

In addition to the conjoint interview assessment, it is also typically useful to conduct a "split" interview, that is, to meet with each spouse alone. During this time potentially sensitive information about each spouse's perception of the marriage can be obtained. In addition, several other issues that may impact substantially on the course of therapy can be clarified.


VERY LOW MARITAL COMMITMENT

An important area to assess before beginning a course of marital therapy is the level of commitment of each spouse to the therapy process as well as to the marriage itself (cf. Stuart, 1980; Beach & Broderick, 1983). In our experience, couples presenting with simultaneous marital discord and depression are particularly difficult to work with if one or both spouses express especially low commitment to work on the marriage. These are cases in which one spouse may state 0 commitment to

# TABLE 4-2. Dyadic Adjustment Scale

| | Always agree | Almost always agree | Occasionally disagree | Frequently disagree | Almost always disagree | Always disagree |
|---|---|---|---|---|---|---|
| 1. Handling family finances | 5 | 4 | 3 | 2 | 1 | 0 |
| 2. Matters of recreation | 5 | 4 | 3 | 2 | 1 | 0 |
| 3. Religious matters | 5 | 4 | 3 | 2 | 1 | 0 |
| 4. Demonstrations of affection | 5 | 4 | 3 | 2 | 1 | 0 |
| 5. Friends | 5 | 4 | 3 | 2 | 1 | 0 |
| 6. Sex relations | 5 | 4 | 3 | 2 | 1 | 0 |
| 7. Conventionality (correct or proper behavior) | 5 | 4 | 3 | 2 | 1 | 0 |
| 8. Philosophy of life | 5 | 4 | 3 | 2 | 1 | 0 |
| 9. Ways of dealing with parents or in-laws | 5 | 4 | 3 | 2 | 1 | 0 |
| 10. Aims, goals, and things believed important | 5 | 4 | 3 | 2 | 1 | 0 |
| 11. Amount of time spent together | 5 | 4 | 3 | 2 | 1 | 0 |
| 12. Making major decisions | 5 | 4 | 3 | 2 | 1 | 0 |
| 13. Household tasks | 5 | 4 | 3 | 2 | 1 | 0 |
| 14. Leisure-time interests and activities | 5 | 4 | 3 | 2 | 1 | 0 |
| 15. Career decisions | 5 | 4 | 3 | 2 | 1 | 0 |

| | All the time | Most of the time | More often than not | Occasionally | Rarely | Never |
|---|---|---|---|---|---|---|
| 16. How often do you discuss or have you considered divorce, separation, or terminating your relationship? | 0 | 1 | 2 | 3 | 4 | 5 |
| 17. How often do you or your mate leave the house after a fight? | 0 | 1 | 2 | 3 | 4 | 5 |
| 18. In general, how often do you think that things between you and your partner are going well? | 5 | 4 | 3 | 2 | 1 | 0 |
| 19. Do you confide in your mate? | 5 | 4 | 3 | 2 | 1 | 0 |
| 20. Do you ever regret that you married (or lived together)? | 0 | 1 | 2 | 3 | 4 | 5 |
| 21. How often do you and your partner quarrel? | 0 | 1 | 2 | 3 | 4 | 5 |
| 22. How often do you and your mate "get on each other's nerves"? | 0 | 1 | 2 | 3 | 4 | 5 |

23. Do you kiss your mate?

| Every day | Almost every day | Occasionally | Rarely | Never |
|---|---|---|---|---|
| 4 | 3 | 2 | 1 | 0 |

24. Do you and your mate engage in outside interests together?

| All of them | Most of them | Some of them | Very few of them | None of them |
|---|---|---|---|---|
| 4 | 3 | 2 | 1 | 0 |

How often would you say the following occur between you and your mate:

| | Never | Less than once a month | Once or twice a month | Once or twice a week | Once a day | More often |
|---|---|---|---|---|---|---|
| 25. Have a stimulating exchange of ideas | 0 | 1 | 2 | 3 | 4 | 5 |
| 26. Laugh together | 0 | 1 | 2 | 3 | 4 | 5 |
| 27. Calmly discuss something | 0 | 1 | 2 | 3 | 4 | 5 |
| 28. Work together on a project | 0 | 1 | 2 | 3 | 4 | 5 |

These are some things about which couples sometimes agree and sometimes disagree. Indicate if either item below caused differences of opinions or were problems in your relationship during the past few weeks. (Check yes or no.)

| | Yes | No | |
|---|---|---|---|
| 29. | 0 | 1 | Being too tired for sex |
| 30. | 0 | 1 | Not showing love |

31. The dots on the following line represent different degrees of happiness in your relationship. The point, "happy," represents the degree of happiness of most relationships. Please circle the dot that best describes the degree of happiness, all things considered, of your relationship.

| 0 | 1 | 2 | 3 | 4 | 5 | 6 |
|---|---|---|---|---|---|---|
| Extremely unhappy | Fairly unhappy | A little unhappy | Happy | Very happy | Extremely happy | Perfect |

32. Which of the following statements best describes how you feel about the future of your relationship:

5  I want desperately for my relationship to succeed and would go to almost any lengths to see that it does.
4  I want very much for my relationship to succeed and will do all that I can to see that it does.
3  I want very much for my relationship to succeed and will do my fair share to see that it does.
2  It would be nice if my relationship succeeded, and I can't do much more than I am doing now to help it succeed.
1  It would be nice if it succeeded, but I refuse to do any more than I am doing now to keep the relationship going.
0  My relationship can never succeed, and there is no more that I can do to keep the relationship going.

Note. From Spanier, G. B. (1976). Measuring dyad adjustment: New scales for assessing the quality of marriage and similar dyads. Journal of Marriage and the Family, 38, 15–28. Copyright 1976 by the National Council on Family Relations. Reprinted by permission of the publisher and author.

work on the relationship in response to the Broderick Commitment Scale (Table 4-3).

This type of response is often an open declaration of an unwillingness to work in therapy, at least initially. This typically predicts lowered compliance with therapist directives, which in turn leads to poorer outcome (Beach & Broderick, 1983). Since the presence of depression tends to exacerbate frustration and tendencies to give up in response to initial failures, we have found that depressed patients expressing very low commitment are more likely than their nondepressed counterparts to conclude that their marriages are hopeless on the basis of an initial failure experience in therapy. These couples may exit precipitously from the marital therapy process. Accordingly, when couples present with extremely low levels of commitment we recommend that the therapist begin with individual therapy for depression.

Interestingly, it has been our experience that couples in which the depressed spouse reports thoughts of divorce may do well in marital therapy as long as expressed commitment to the marriage remains high. Thus serious consideration of divorce need not get in the way of working on marital issues with the depressed, discordant couple.


## HIDDEN AGENDAS

Sometimes persons presenting for marital therapy initially report that they wish to work on their marriage when in actuality they have already decided to terminate the relationship as soon as possible. In some cases the nondepressed spouse may use marital therapy to create a convenient time to exit the relationship, announcing after one or two sessions the plan to leave that was made months earlier. In other cases it may be the depressed spouse who has already decided that the marriage is unworkable but feels compelled to "go through the motions" of therapy in order to demonstrate that every effort was made; only later in therapy is it discovered that separation was actually the preferred outcome of therapy. Hidden agendas are disruptive of therapy by their very nature. In essence, the therapist mistakenly believes that a collaborative relationship is about to emerge when this is not, in fact, going to happen.

In order to deal with the possibility of hidden agendas, couples are specifically asked during the individual interviews about any interest in leaving the marriage. It is explained that marital therapy requires an initial investment that is fairly substantial in terms of both time and energy. Thus they are allowed to express any reservations they might have about expending this time and effort in order to help improve their marriage and possibly aid their spouse. While this procedure does have

TABLE 4-3. Broderick Commitment Scale

Commitment can be viewed as the degree to which an individual is willing to stand by another even though that may mean putting aside one's own needs and desires for the sake of the other; it can mean a time of accepting the other person in spite of his/her faults or problems that may make one's own life more difficult; it can mean thinking less about the immediate advantages and disadvantages of the relationship and working to make the relationship last in the long run.

Given this description, select a number from the scale below to indicate how "committed" you are to your marriage.

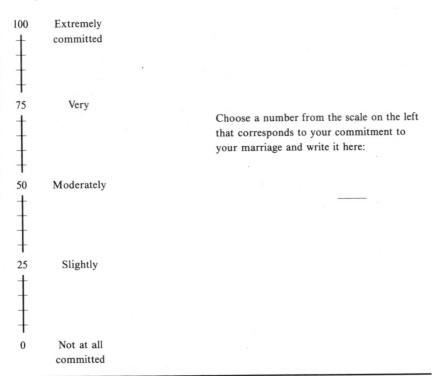

100  Extremely
     committed

75   Very

     Choose a number from the scale on the left
     that corresponds to your commitment to
     your marriage and write it here:

50   Moderately

     _____

25   Slightly

0    Not at all
     committed

the drawback of occasionally producing secrets that are known only to the therapist and one spouse, we find that this is preferable to having these secrets gradually unfold as a hidden agenda of one spouse later on in therapy. If spouses are able to state that their primary goal is to get out of the marriage with a minimum disruption, this is important information for the marital therapist to have. Standard marital therapy is unlikely to produce changes in the marriage in such cases. Additionally, the therapist is in a position to recommend that individual therapy be offered as an alternative. The spouse wishing to end the relationship can also be encouraged to reveal the "secret" to the depressed patient in an appropriate manner, rather than producing this surprise later in therapy.

## REFUSAL TO STOP EXTRAMARITAL SEX

It is sometimes discovered during a split assessment that one of the spouses has been or is involved in extramarital sexual activity (cf. Beach et al., 1985). Even in marital therapy where the depression of one spouse is not a major concern, this can complicate the therapy considerably, although some forms of marital work may still be viable. However, in our experience, for the depressed and discordant couple the presence of *ongoing* extramarital sexual activity is incompatible with constructive work on relationship issues. This type of activity is incompatible with making the kinds of changes in short-term marital therapy that are likely to be most beneficial for the couple. Gains in closeness, positive time together, intimacy, and openness of communication are particularly compromised if one partner is actively involved in extramarital sexual relations. Accordingly, the therapist should explain in a nonjudgmental manner that there is little point to involving the couple in this type of marital therapy while the extramarital sexual activity continues. If the involved spouse refuses to stop the extramarital relationship, marital therapy for depression is not an appropriate treatment strategy. Marital work may be appropriate later, of course, if the depression is successfully addressed through other means or the extramarital relationship is terminated.

It is often necessary to explain to spouses that extramarital sex is typically not workable in the context of a healthy marriage. Some spouses have retained false information disseminated during the late 1960s and early 1970s suggesting that "swinging" or more open sexual relationships are workable alternatives to traditional monogamous relationships. It is important to point out to these individuals that there is little reason to believe that extramarital sex is in any way compatible with a stable, well-functioning marriage. Spouses involved in extramarital affairs should be encouraged to think in terms of choosing between improving their marital relationship and leaving it, rather than hoping that the situation can continue as it is. The depressed spouse is not necessarily worse off when a decision to terminate the relationship is reached. In some cases this allows an unsettled situation to achieve closure and so facilitates recovery from the depression.

## Process Issues

### Dual Alliance

Both spouses must feel that they have a therapeutic alliance with the marital therapist. If only one spouse feels such an alliance, while the other spouse feels left out, this can lead to serious problems in the ongoing process of therapy. When there is not a dual alliance, it is likely that therapy will break down and yield relatively few positive results. In the context of depression, however, it is extremely tempting for the therapist to establish a differential alliance with the two participants. On the one hand, it may be tempting for the therapist to side with the nondepressed spouse, seeing this partner as the long-suffering and aggrieved party in the relationship. On the other hand, it may be tempting to side with the depressed patient, seeing this partner as a victim of spousal insensitivity. When these temptations arise, it should be remembered that the depressed, discordant couple is really not very different from the nondepressed, discordant couple. There is always more than enough blame to share in dysfunctional relationships, and there are always differing possible perspectives as to how the blame should be divided between the spouses. It is no more difficult for the therapist to maintain the dual alliance in the context of depression than it is in any other marital case.

### Depressive Venting

During the course of marital therapy with depressed patients, there are likely to be occasions when the depressed patient gives vent to a variety of negative feelings, complaints, and expressions of dysphoria. Once begun, these episodes can dominate an entire session. It is our experience that it is not always most helpful to terminate these episodes of venting in a premature fashion. Rather, they can often be incorporated into the ongoing process of therapy, either as an opportunity for the therapist to model active listening or as an opportunity to involve the nondepressed spouse in a caring and reflective listening process. This is often the very material to which the nondepressed spouse finds it most difficult to attend. It may also be the very material the depressed patient feels is least listened to by the spouse. Accordingly, it can be useful material to work with therapeutically.

It is also important to note that attempts to be overstrict with the depressed patient and to bring the couple too quickly back on task can be counterproductive. Under such circumstances, depressed patients are prone to view the remainder of the session as being irrelevant to their primary concerns. Their lack of involvement and attention to the ongoing session is likely to be apparent to both the therapist and the nondepressed spouse. This, in turn, is likely to generate considerable pessimism and frustration on the part of the nondepressed spouse. Thus, by ending depressive venting episodes too quickly, it is possible to precipitate a deteriorating spiral of frustration and pessimism in therapy.

On the other hand, depressive venting can also continue longer than is necessary for purposes of therapy if the therapist is not alert to opportunities to bring the session back to the initially agreed-upon agenda. Thus the therapist must also take the opportunity to reflect back the concerns of the depressed patient, reinforce the spouse for active listening, and suggest that the concerns being expressed can be added to future agendas. In this way the therapist can use the episode for maximal therapeutic benefit while limiting its potential to sidetrack therapy.

## Noncompliance

Noncompliance with the requests of the therapist appears to be associated with poor outcome in marital therapy for depression (Sandeen, O'Leary, & Beach, 1987). In our clinical experience, it appears that episodes of noncompliance can reasonably be subdivided. A nonexhaustive list of reasons for noncompliance would include: (1) episodes that are manifestations of giving up and an underlying pessimism regarding the potential usefulness of marital therapy; (2) episodes that are the result of underlying hidden agendas on the part of one or both spouses (e.g., one spouse wants out of the marriage); (3) episodes in which the noncompliance is an unspoken message to the therapist that the couple is dissatisfied with the assignment; (4) episodes in which the noncompliance results from entrenched control battles between the spouses or episodes of blame and punishment; and (5) the more benign forms of noncompliance that pose relatively little threat to the ongoing integrity of the therapeutic effort.

The first form of noncompliance, giving up, is an extremely important form of noncompliance to recognize and to deal with in a depressed, discordant population. Depressed individuals and their spouses typically have a long history of futile attempts at changing their relationship. As with other maritally discordant couples, their ingrained coercive patterns and exchanges are very automatic, and when they begin to attempt changes they find that their more ingrained reactions quickly resurface. However, depressed, discordant couples appear particularly likely to see a minor obstacle as a reason for giving up. Accordingly, the clinician must be ready to explain that change is not an overnight process. Very subtle forms of change need to be pointed out for the couple, and positive tracking needs to be emphasized. The primary concern of the therapist when dealing with this type of noncompliance is to help prevent a premature termination of efforts to work on the marriage.

The second form of noncompliance, that involving hidden agendas, is also extremely serious. This is most often seen when one spouse appears to be doing far less than can be explained on the basis of ability and stated intention. Most often, noncompliant spouses will blame their partners for not doing their part in order to justify failure to complete their own portion of the assigned homework. One response to this behavior is to address the separate and individual responsibility of each partner to complete his/her portion of the assigned homework despite the behavior of the other partner. However, when a hidden agenda is active, this type of explanation is unlikely to have any impact. Following repeated examples of such behavior, we believe it is appropriate to have a split session in which another round of assessment is done and the behavior is explored in detail with the apparently offending partner.

A third form of noncompliance can arise when the couple feels that therapy is off track or one spouse feels that the therapist has allied with the other spouse against him/her. This form of noncompliance is very important to explore, since it potentially holds the answer to successful change with the couple or represents the first stage in the collapse of therapy. Dealing with this type of noncompliance requires a nonjudgmental and open exploration of the couple's thoughts and feelings surrounding the homework. Not only does this form of noncompliance not need to lead to problems in the course of therapy; it can actually be quite helpful. It can allow the clinician to show openness to feedback and a willingness to work in a truly collaborative mode. In addition to its benefit for the therapeutic alliance with the dyad, this type of exchange can also model a nondefensive way of dealing with criticism and provide the clinician with an opportunity to reinforce the open expression of thoughts and concerns. Thus the clinician's response to noncompliance resulting from dissatisfaction can be very usefully incorporated into the ongoing therapy.

A fourth type of noncompliance appears to result from overlearned, rapidly escalating negative interactions. These interactions may lead couples to engage in behavior they had agreed to avoid, such as violence or name calling. This type of noncompliance is probably best dealt with through a combination of reiterating the directions previously given, noting the difficulty in changing such behaviors, and exploring the possible thoughts or situational determinants that led to the rapid escalation.

To the extent that particular situations or thoughts that trigger these exchanges can be found, assignments may be embellished to maximize opportunity for success. In particular, it is likely that blame and feeling that the partner deserves to be punished will emerge as important determinants of this type of noncompliance. Accordingly, it may be necessary to explore the basis of these attributions of blame and to help each partner find new ways of understanding the other's behavior before marital therapy can proceed successfully.

The fifth form of noncompliance is the relatively random periods of noncompliance that seem to occur in the course of virtually all therapy. In this form of noncompliance, clients do not do some type of therapeutic assignment because they have decided as a couple that they do not wish to do it, or because they find something better to do, or because they misunderstand something about the assignment itself. In these cases, it is often possible to reinterpret the response to the assignment in a positive light and point to the gains that were made in any case. Since making gains is the point of the therapeutic process, the failure to complete a particular therapeutic assignment can be presented as being of minimal importance.

## Managing Suicidal Threats and Threats of Separation

During the course of marital therapy it is possible that acute stressors will arise that prompt suicidal threats on the part of the depressed patient or threats of separation by either partner. These threats need to be dealt with in a forthright manner. We find that suicidal threats are better dealt with in an individual format. Accordingly, when suicidal threats are presented we take a break in marital therapy and begin an individual focus on the suicidal ideation and the direct alleviation of depressed symptomatology. When threats of separation are presented, it is important to explore them in detail to determine their apparent origin. If they represent a relatively stable, well-thought-out intention on the part of one spouse, then appropriate steps must be taken to prepare for marital dissolution. Conversely, if it appears that the threat of separation is being used as a form of marital communication and does not represent a stable, well-formed intention, then this can be dealt with in the overall context of marital therapy.

The maladaptive and coercive nature of using threats of marital separation needs to be explored, as well as alternative ways of approaching problem solving. Thus such behavior can be discussed as merely one of a large variety of behaviors that occur in the context of marital discord. In addition, the partner using the threat can be instructed to use alternative and less destructive means of making his/her point.

## The Therapist's Role in Marital Therapy for Depression

Stuart (1980) delineates five dimensions of the therapist's role in marital therapy: administration, mediation, reeducation, modeling, and celebrating. Within these dimensions, the therapist doing marital therapy with depressed spouses must always be sensitive to issues of depression as well as marital dynamics. Following are our suggestions on how the therapist can best fulfill his/her role demands with this population.

## Administration

As the administrator of the therapy, the therapist must pay attention to details of planning treatment sessions and setting goals (in collaboration with the couple). The therapist should always set an agenda for the session, share that agenda with the clients at the beginning of the session, and ask for feedback about the adequacy of the agenda. The therapist is then responsible for using therapeutic time wisely and for pacing its content over both the individual session and the entire course of therapy.

The administrative role requires the therapist to perform a delicate balancing act between structure and flexibility. Depressed clients need and appreciate structure in their marital therapy sessions; structure helps dispel the feeling of hopelessness and instills confidence in the therapist's abilities. On the other hand, the therapist must explicitly attempt to elicit feedback from the couple (especially from the depressed individuals) in regard to how adequately the structure provided meets their needs. Depressed clients may tend to be unassertive in telling the therapist they have a problem that needs to be addressed in therapy, if it is not on the therapist's planned agenda for that session (cf. Beck et al., 1979).

As the administrator, the therapist also has to skillfully make the therapeutic model relevant for each particular couple. For example, the therapist is responsible for deciding on homework assignments that both fulfill the goals of the model and are meaningful for each particular couple. Homework assignments must emerge from the problems and strengths of the couple; they cannot be decided on in detail *a priori*.

## Mediation

As a mediator, the therapist must create a therapeutic alliance with the clients *as a couple*. The therapeutic stance must be one of neutrality in relation to the two partners. The therapist will often be asked to judge who is right in a given instance, but the role of judge should typically be rejected by the therapist. Instead, the correct role of the therapist is to help the couple express themselves clearly to each other and to come to solutions to their problems that are mutually agreeable. Alliances with individuals within the couple are nonproductive and countertherapeutic. Even if it appears that one partner is "the bad one," it is imperative that the therapist not form an alliance with one partner against the other. The therapist must be vigilant that there is not even the perception of favoritism toward one partner. Thus we attempt to make all interventions and in-session feedback symmetrical with regard to the two clients; that is, if one partner is given critical feedback or a homework assignment directed at behavior change, the other should also be given feedback or homework.

## Reeducation

Much of what the therapist does can be considered reeducation. As a reeducator of depressed persons, it is important that the therapist communicate the reasonableness of the clients' previous beliefs regarding marriage and depression while at the same time introducing them to new beliefs and skills. For example, at various points throughout therapy it will be important to indicate to the depressed patient that many things are contributing to the depression, that being depressed makes it difficult to initiate changes in behavior patterns, and that things will not feel as good as they would if he/she were not depressed. It is also likely to be important to point out that loss of sexual desire is a common symptom of depression and that such desire may not return until very late in the recovery process. In each case, the therapist attempts to substitute more accurate information for information that is inaccurate and likely to cause problems.

## Modeling

The therapist plays an important role in providing a calm, problem-oriented model for the clients. Additionally, the therapist will explicitly model particular skills as a teaching device. Obviously, if the therapist is not able to remain calm and unruffled in the face of the clients' problems, he/she cannot adequately demonstrate the interpersonal skills the clients need to see. It can be upsetting for the therapist to deal with clients presenting with both marital discord and depression. They are frequently "difficult" clients. However, the therapist must be aware that he/she is constantly "on display" for the clients and is always teaching something via his/her behavior. The therapist should make every effort to teach only what is therapeutic for the couple.

## Celebrating

In the role of celebrant, the therapist functions as a reinforcer of positive changes. Real gains and positive changes are often overlooked by clients. The therapist, however, acknowledges positive change and helps the couple notice and feel good about their new behaviors. In this capacity, the therapist is also lending an official stamp of approval to changes in the couple's life. Depressed clients especially need to be encouraged to feel good about changes they have made, since their tendency may be to discount small improvements (cf. Beck et al., 1979). It is in this role that the therapist can also interject humor and a compassionate yet cheerful attitude toward life. It is particularly important for the therapist to help couples gradually share this role by noticing, complimenting, thanking, and commenting on desired positive changes. Depressed and discordant couples will usually not display good ability to notice small changes and reinforce these changes in each other. Thus, by taking on the role of celebrant, the therapist models this skill for both spouses. It also follows from this perspective that homework assignments should be designed to maximize opportunities to celebrate with the couple. One strategy is to very carefully gradate assignments, as is often done in individual therapy for depression. Indeed, this is really little more than creatively assigning successive approximations that lead step by step to a large change in the marital environment.

## What Marital Therapy for Depression Is Not

One possible way of dealing with relationship difficulties that occur in tandem with a depressive episode is to use an essentially individual therapy approach but to involve the spouse in therapy in some manner. For example, Beck discussed the possibility of training the spouse to be an ally in the therapeutic process. In this approach, the spouse would serve as an "auxiliary therapist" who could help implement therapeutic strategies in the home situation (Beck et al., 1979). This notion has been further elaborated by Rush, Shaw, and Khatami (1980). In this approach, the involvement of the spouse does not attempt to address destructive relationship processes that may be contributing to or maintaining the episode of depression; rather, the involvement of the spouse is seen as a potentially positive influence on the normal course of individual therapy. For depressed couples who are nondiscordant or very mildly discordant, we suspect that spousal involvement along the lines suggested in these proposals can, at times, be quite beneficial. However, for discordant, depressed couples we view these speculations with some alarm. In our experience with discordant, depressed couples, the nondepressed spouse can hardly be considered a neutral observer of ongoing marital events. More typically, the nondepressed spouse is overcritical, often behaves in an unaccepting and nonempathic manner, and is actively contributing his/her share to the ongoing marital discord. This is hardly the ideal image of an auxiliary therapist. If we attempt to make the spouse an auxiliary therapist while he/she is still actively contributing to the marital discord, that spouse is more likely to be a destructive influence than a helpful addition to therapy.

An additional constraint on the use of spouses as auxiliary therapists in dealing with depressed, discordant patients is the hesitancy of patients to allow their spouses to assume such a role. We find this hesitancy entirely understandable. The depressed spouse may be concerned about disclosing hostile thoughts directed toward the partner. The discomfort of this situation is compounded when only the depressed spouse is expected to self-disclose. In the absence of a solid, trusting, nondiscordant marital relationship, the task being assigned to the depressed patient in such a therapeutic arrangement is a difficult task indeed.

Our own perspective is that marital therapy that directly addresses and corrects the destructive interactions in the relationship is required before the nondepressed spouse is in a position to act as an auxiliary therapist; that is, in the context of ongoing marital discord, marital therapy is likely to be necessary before the nondepressed spouse can be used to facilitate some other individually oriented therapy process. True marital therapy recognizes the nondepressed spouse as an equal participant in the relationship difficulties that have emerged. Thus, beginning with marital therapy allows the nondepressed spouse to correct those interactional patterns that he/she has been contributing to the relationship dysfunction. Once this task has been completed, and the nondepressed spouse has been socialized into therapy as an equal rather than as a superior to the depressed partner, he/she is much more likely to make helpful and insightful remarks about the depressed spouse and the recovery process. In our experience, however, when marital therapy is successfully completed, the depressive episode often remits as well. Accordingly, when the clinician is faced with ongoing marital discord along with depression, it will often make sense to directly address dysfunctional relationship patterns first. We have found that further therapy for depression is often not required.

## A Session-by-Session Outline of Marital Therapy for Depression

It is sometimes helpful to have a schematic illustration of a "typical course of therapy." This outline is presented for heuristic reasons only. In practice, this outline should not be adhered to rigidly, since each couple will bring their own limitations, special concerns, and crises to therapy. In addition, the models approach to therapy explicitly calls for the therapist to be willing to tailor the therapy to each client and apply techniques in a clinically flexible manner. It is common for couples to learn one or another skill less quickly than the outline would lead one to believe. For each particular couple the skill requiring additional time may be different. Rather than push ahead when a particular skill is not yet well learned or a particular issue is not yet resolved, it makes more sense to move forward in therapy as is indicated clinically. Some couples may benefit from a longer course of therapy than the one outlined below, and therapists should not hesitate to extend therapy when indicated. Alternatively, some couples may not show problems in the usual areas, and therapy may then proceed more rapidly than usual. In every case the needs of the couple should be evaluated relative to the relationship skills and activities that the marital discord model highlights as being necessary for their long-term ability to remain nondiscordant and nondepressed. The details of how to apply particular techniques to a depressed, discordant client population are articulated in Chapters 5 through 7. Skills and homework assignments for sessions 2–4 are described in detail in Chapter 5; those for sessions 5–11 are found in Chapter 6. In addition, specific and general skills important in the application of marital therapy for depression are outlined in the Appendix. In the session-by-session outline below, it is assumed that an initial assessment has already been conducted.

## Session 1

1. Set the agenda for the session with the couple, including concerns they want to discuss.

2. Briefly review assessment information. For example, "I see from your assessment packet that you agree that the major problems right now center on difficulties with anger and arguing." Never disclose particular information from one partner's written assessment material without his/her approval.

3. Give the couple information on the nature of depression (see Chapter 1).

4. Give the couple some information on the treatment model under which you are operating. For example, "We know that marital problems and feelings of depression are often related to each other. This happens either because the marital problems themselves create stress and turmoil and so lead to depression, or else because the marriage has trouble adapting to times when one person is depressed and so doesn't play as active and positive a role as it potentially can in helping alleviate the depression. So we will be focusing here on working directly to help the marriage play as active and positive a role as it can in helping reduce negative feelings and increase positive feelings."

5. Take information on the history of the relationship, the problems within the relationship, and the strengths of the relationship. The focus should be positive by the end of the assessment if at all possible; for example, identifying things that attracted them to each other, describing current problems as decreases in the positive things they once had.

6. Summarize what was done in this session and make a tentative agreement with the couple on which problems will be worked on in therapy. End on a positive and hopeful note.


## Session 2

1. Set the agenda with the couple.

2. Gather information on ways that the couple currently expresses love and caring to each other and on their individual and joint positive activities. Reinforce with positive attention any signs, however small, of positive change.

3. Explain homework assignment of "caring days" to couple and begin to generate caring menu in session.

4. Explore the existence of very negative behaviors in the couple (e.g., verbal or physical abuse, threats to leave the relationship, examarital affairs). If these are ongoing, the session must be devoted to discussion of the consequences of such behaviors, and treatment directed at stopping these must take priority over other treatment.

5. Summarize the session and give homework assignment of completing caring menu at home or beginning caring gestures (depending on how far the couple gets in session). Homework may also include increasing positive individual time if one partner is quite depressed and is having little rewarding activity. End on a positive and hopeful note.

## Session 3

1. Set the agenda with the couple. Ask about positive couple activities.

2. Go over the homework assignment. If the assignment was not completed, discuss this as a problem to be solved for next week. Praise any effort, and turn the assignment into a learning experience for the couple.

3. Explore in more detail what joint activities the couple would find pleasant. Try to pick one or two and discuss them in detail, with an eye to choosing an activity that looks like it will lead to a pleasant experience.

4. Summarize the session and give homework assignment of continuing caring gestures from the menu and also planning and carrying out at least one joint activity. Point out any pattern of positive change in the relationship. Help spouses compliment each other.

## Session 4

1. Set the agenda with the couple. Ask about positive couple activities.

2. Go over the homework assignment. Attend to problems in completing the assignment and praise improvements and attempts at change. Emphasize the improvement in feelings that came from a successful attempt at changing their behavior with each other.

3. Introduce communication training. Collateral readings (e.g., Gottman, Notarius, Gonso, & Markman, 1979) may be used.

4. Have the couple listen to themselves in taped interaction of the two of them. Have them comment on their own communication. Emphasize a focus on changing oneself.

5. Summarize the session and give assignment of continuing with positive joint activities and caring days. Also, assign readings on communication and ask each partner to monitor his/her own communication during the week (not change it, simply monitor it). Help spouses pat themselves on the back for their changes.

## Session 5

1. Set the agenda with the couple. Ask about positive couple activities.

2. Go over assignments. Emphasize any positive benefit of changing one's behavior, and emphasize changes the couple has made since the beginning of therapy. Address difficulties the couple may have had in completing the assignments. Reinforce with positive attention any effort in completing the assignments. Reflect on all that has been learned and how it seems to have already reduced feelings of depression and increased positive interactions in the marriage.

3. Introduce listener skills and practice of listener skills with the couple.

4. Summarize the session and give assignment of using listener skills in a 5-minute discussion at home, which is to be audiotaped and brought into the next session. The topic for discussion should not be a marital problem. Point out continuing positive changes in the dyad.

## Session 6

1. Set the agenda with the couple. Ask about positive couple activities.

2. Play the assignment tape and have each member of the couple criticize their own performance of listener skills. Guide the critique and give your own critique of the tape. Provide praise, dwell on areas of strength, and point out what is being done well.

3. Continue with listener skill introduction and practice.

4. Summarize the session and give assignment to use these new skills in a tape-recorded session at home. The topic of discussion should not be a marital problem area, and it should be chosen in discussion with you. Reflect on gains in therapy.

## Session 7

1. Set the agenda with the couple. Ask about positive couple activities.

2. Play the assignment tape and discuss the strengths and problems of the communication.

3. Introduce speaker skills and practice with the couple.

4. Summarize the session and give assignment to use new skills in tape-recorded session at home. Clients can pick the topic, which can

include low-level marital problems but should stay away from very explosive ones. Reflect on gains in therapy.

## Session 8

1. Set the agenda with the couple. Ask about positive couple activities.
2. Play the assignment tape and discuss the strengths and problems of the communication.
3. Continue with speaker skill introduction and practice.
4. Summarize the session and give assignment to use new skills in tape-recorded session at home. It may be time to attempt exploration of a somewhat more difficult problem area.
5. Discuss the increasing strength of the relationship.

## Session 9

1. Set the agenda with the couple. Ask about positive couple activities.
2. Play the assignment tape and discuss it.
3. Introduce problem solving and practice the skill in session, using a small problem or a nonexistent "practice" problem.
4. Summarize the session and give assignment of using problem solving during a tape-recorded session at home. You should help the couple pick a "small" topic. Help them pat themselves on the back.

## Session 10

1. Set the agenda with the couple. Ask about positive couple activities.
2. Play the assignment tape and discuss it.
3. Continue with problem-solving practice in session.
4. Summarize the session and give assignment of using problem solving during a tape-recorded session at home. The couple may pick the topic. Praise couple progress and reflect on their enhanced feelings of openness.

## Session 11

1. Set the agenda with the couple. Ask about positive couple activities.

2. Play the assignment tape and discuss it.

3. Have the couple use problem-solving skills in session to discuss problems in the relationship that they feel have not been resolved thus far.

4. Summarize the session and have the couple continue the problem-solving discussion at home. If you are confident of the couple's communication skills, it need not be tape-recorded. Otherwise, it should be taped so it can be analyzed next session. Praise couple progress.

## Session 12

1. Set the agenda with the couple. Ask about positive couple activities.

2. Play the assignment tape or discuss the homework assignment. Problem solve about what could be done differently if the home session went poorly.

3. Introduce the topic of termination of therapy. Elicit fears and concerns about the subject.

4. Summarize the session and have the couple design their own homework assignment, one that addresses a problem currently concerning them. Have the couple praise each other on their couple progress.

## Session 13

1. Set the agenda with the couple.

2. Review different interventions tried during therapy and discuss what was helpful and not helpful for them, and why.

3. Summarize the session and have the couple design their own homework assignment, one that uses a technique they previously used in therapy but have stopped using. Praise the couple on their ability to face new challenges on their own.

## Session 14

1. Set the agenda with the couple.

2. Continue the review of interventions from the previous session. Practice techniques the couple does not feel sure of.

3. Summarize the session and have the couple design their own homework assignment.

## Session 15

1. Set the agenda with the couple.

2. Engage in trouble-shooting regarding what could go wrong to make them lose the gains made in therapy. Problem solve regarding how to maintain gains.

3. Discuss the inevitability of ups and downs in marital satisfaction and warn against the tendency to see a temporary downswing as an irreversible change in the relationship or as evidence that nothing has really changed in the marriage.

4. Summarize the session and make an appointment for a "booster" session.

# 5

## The Initial Phase of Therapy: Gaining Momentum for Positive Change

Once the assessments have been completed and a decision has been reached that marital intervention would be appropriate with a particular depressed couple, it is appropriate to intervene rapidly for the purposes of: (1) increasing marital cohesion and associated displays of affection, (2) increasing self-esteem and marital support, and (3) reducing or eliminating severe, recurrent marital stressors. This chapter will present the treatment strategy and techniques we employ most typically during this first phase of marital therapy for depression. The first phase of therapy typically will last three to five sessions. Therapy techniques we have used to fulfill the three primary goals of this phase of therapy will be described in sufficient detail to allow persons with only beginning marital therapy experience to understand the basic elements involved. However, it should be understood that *any* technique that produces changes in the areas of the marital relationship highlighted by the marital discord model should be a potentially useful tool in the treatment of co-occurring marital discord and depression. Finally, a number of issues that play an important role during this initial phase of therapy will be discussed.

### Increasing Marital Cohesion

Couples presenting with the joint problems of marital discord and depression appear to be particularly likely to show low levels of couple cohesion (Beach, Nelson, & O'Leary, 1988). Thus, these couples tend to be low in the type of shared positive activity one might expect to have antidepressant properties (Lewinsohn & Arconad, 1981). By addressing cohesion early in therapy, the therapist is attempting to bring about a rapid shift in the amount of positive, enjoyable time spent together by the couple and increase the rate of positive exchange and ongoing displays of affection. The techniques most appropriate for this goal are drawn from the pool of support–understanding strategies currently available to marital therapists (Weiss, 1978). These strategies are particularly useful for the depressed and discordant couple, because they are designed to reverse the cycle of coercion and withdrawal exhibited prominently by these couples and to reintroduce fun and mutual involvement.

## Caring Gestures

One of the most valuable techniques in the therapist's armamentarium for enhancing the deteriorated cohesion of the depressed, discordant couple is the prescription of increased caring gestures (Stuart, 1980; Weiss & Birchler, 1978), or "couple pleases" and companionship activities (Jacobson & Margolin, 1979). Caring gestures and "couple pleases" focus on mutual relationship pleasures that the spouses agree on. Caring gestures are any behaviors that are designed to please the partner and, in so doing, indicate love and caring. The behaviors to be increased should already be within the response repertoire of the spouses; that is, no new learning should be required in this phase. Also, they are typically rather small actions that could be repeated often. The goal of a caring-gestures focus in therapy is to increase the frequency of already learned responses that are readily available but currently underused. Similarly, companionship activities are joint activities that are enjoyable or have been enjoyable for the couple in the past. Companionship activities are typically somewhat larger actions than caring gestures, possibly involving such activities as going on a date or talking about each other's day. Once again, however, they should be relatively simple and not require new learning.

We typically introduce the topic of caring and companionship by noting the evidence that the spouses care for each other and want to resolve problems and have a more satisfying relationship. This can be challenging at times, but the therapist who cannot make this case at all plausible probably should not be doing marital therapy for depression. Having made the case that at times the spouses exhibit genuine caring impulses and positive feelings toward each other, we then note that many of the day-to-day things that help convey these feelings have disappeared from the relationship. Often one of the partners has commented on this point in the initial interview, and we mention their desire to increase these aspects of the marriage. Thus we immediately set the stage for putting these items on the agenda for the session and continue the agenda-building process with these items as the primary focus of the session. If the agenda building continues uneventfully, we begin intervention promptly. We commonly provide additional rationales for caring items, making sure the rationales make sense to each partner as we begin work in this area. Rationales such as the following may be helpful: "Engaging in reassuring and pleasant interactions is an important first step toward resolving problems. Showing caring for one's spouse also feels good once it is reestablished and feels spontaneous and natural again. In addition, showing caring gives us an opportunity to learn skills in a positive context that will be useful later in therapy as we address problem solving and problem resolution." A rationale of this type helps depressed and discordant couples see more clearly the integrated, cumulative nature of their therapy program and seems to inspire additional hope. It also provides an opportunity for the therapist to prevent the clients from seeing caring items either as the linchpin of their marital relationship or as a sidetrack away from more important issues. Both the overvaluation and the devaluation of caring items can be a problem in therapy, and helping clients understand and accept a rationale that places increased caring and companionship activities in context is central in preventing problems from arising later in therapy.

There are many ways to implement the strategy of increasing caring and companionship behaviors (Jacobson & Margolin, 1979; Liberman, Wheeler, deVisser, Kuehnel, & Kuehnel, 1980; Stuart, 1980). All approaches provide guidance to help the couple better identify, prompt, recognize, and reinforce potentially positive couple behavior. At the very outset, correct identification of pleasing behavior is necesary. It is quite common for couples to have very poor skills in recognizing concrete events that are pleasing or displeasing to one another. Accordingly, they will find that something that one of them thought the other liked is not actually pleasing for that spouse. Thus part of increasing caring behavior is increasing couples "objectification" skills (Weiss, 1978). In one case we saw, the depressed wife finally told her husband that she really did not enjoy it when he brought her roses, because she liked other flowers much better. In fact, she experienced receiving roses from him as a negative event, because it indicated his lack of sensitivity to her preferences. The husband was unaware of his wife's true feelings on this. He had believed that she protested against roses because she thought them too expensive. He therefore viewed giving her roses as showing his great degree of caring for her, despite the expense. Obviously, without identifying what gestures would be positive for the wife, this husband would not have succeeded in showing his caring for her. In another case, both spouses resisted caring-gestures assignments because they did not like the experience of having something done for them. Both members of the couple felt uncomfortable with "owing" anything to anyone, including their partner. Because this was an attitude that was not assessed before the assignment was given, they had a negative experience in attempting to do the assignment. In effect, any "positive" gesture was experienced as an unpleasant event. They were more successful with attempting companionship activities. Later in therapy, increasing caring items was more successful. This illustrates the point that in conducting marital therapy for depression, we try to begin with behaviors that are readily available to the couple. Later in therapy we attempt to build in activities that may require new learning.

Because of the potential for a "positive" gesture's not having the impact intended, we have each spouse individually generate a list of small gestures he/she would like to have the partner perform. We stress to the couple that in compiling such lists, they are not creating a series of demands for their partners. This is important because it prevents the caring list from becoming yet another annoyance or perceived stressor in the relationship. Instead, the lists are to be viewed as menus from which the partner can choose when desirous of performing a caring gesture for his/her mate.

It is also important that the gestures involve *small* behaviors that require no new learning on the part of the partner, that are specific, and that involve increases in positive behavior rather than decreases in negative behavior. "Buying me a new car," for example, would be rejected as an item on a caring-gesture menu, because it involves too large an expenditure of money to be classified as a simple gesture. "Being more sociable at parties" would also be rejected, both because it is too vague and because it may call for new behavior not already within the partner's repertoire. "Stop bothering me when I get home from work" might be included if reworked into "Give me 10 minutes when I get home from work before discussing anything." Better yet would be to rework this item into something more positive, such as "Give me 10 minutes to relax when I get home from work, then bring me a beer (or a soda) and sit down with me." This reworking from a request for an absence of negative behavior to a request for an increase of a positive behavior is important, because the absence of behavior is not usually a salient event. Caring gestures must be salient to both the giver and the receiver in order to be effective. In some cases, a request for a decrease in or elimination of a behavior can be made salient by having the giver label his/her action as a caring gesture. For example, a wife whose husband requests time alone when he gets home could say to him on his arrival, "Hi, honey, go on into the den and relax for a while. I got the kids to play at Jeanne's so you can unwind alone until 6:30." In this way, she is making salient her effort in arranging for her husband's quiet time alone. The saliency also allows the husband to acknowledge her gesture.

Especially encouraged on caring-gesture menus are gestures that can be performed frequently, that call for minimal monetary expenditure, and that are under the giver's total control. These guidelines are all designed to prevent the problems couples frequently have in carrying out the assignment to perform caring gestures. Gestures that are too expensive or too time consuming, or that depend on some outside circumstance to come about, are unlikely to be performed (or will be performed infrequently). Thus we encourage caring lists that include such things as giving backrubs, sending love notes, making unexpected phone calls, giving compliments, fixing a favorite snack, bringing home a small surprise, and doing a chore for the other person. (There are many good ideas for such gestures in the "fun deck" and "up deck" appendices in Gottman, Notarius, Gonso, & Markman, 1976.) Particularly with a depressed, discordant couple, the therapist should anticipate spending time with the couple generating possible items for each list. It is not uncommon for spouses in the depressed, discordant couples to initially have trouble thinking of even one small thing that their partner could do for them. We have found it helpful to point out that if this is a difficult activity for them to do for themselves, then it should come as no surprise that it is difficult for their partner, who (1) cannot read their mind and (2) cannot do it without their guidance and input. This observation uses their own frustration with generating items to help reduce anger toward and blame of the spouse for not doing more for them. However, the therapist should not let couples suffer too long before making a few suggestions to get the ball rolling (see sample caring-gesture list in Table 5-1, below). Depressed and discordant couples do not typically deal well with frustration in therapy, and so frustrating experiences should be rationed carefully.

After identification of positive events is accomplished, some type of prompting for increased exchange of caring behavior is typically necessary. In this regard, we have found that three aspects of the caring assignment are essential for depressed and discordant couples: (1) emphasizing that the caring gestures should be performed *daily*; (2) emphasizing that each spouse is responsible for performing caring gestures for the partner *independently* of the partner's success in performing caring gestures for him/her; (3) emphasizing the importance of giving recognition when caring gestures have been performed. The rationale given to the couple for making the assignment a daily one is that caring gestures are supposed to be small indications of underlying feeling and, as such, need to be given generously in order to effectively demonstrate positive feeling. However, it is also the case that depressed persons show a very consistent tendency to underestimate the rate of positives they experience and to have some difficulty recalling positive experiences (DeMonbreun & Craighead, 1977). Accordingly, for the depressed spouse anything below a frequency of several gestures daily may be too infrequent to be observed and recalled.

The independence of the assignments given to husband and wife is designed to help couples out of the common pattern of "tit for tat"— "Why should I do something nice when he/she hasn't?" It has been found that while satisfied couples do not require immediate reciprocation of positive and negative interactions, dissatisfied couples display a more "tit for tat" interaction style, in which they tend to reciprocate what their partner has just done to them (Gottman, 1979, 1980; Notarius et al., 1989). Also, evidence is mounting that this interactional style can predict subsequent deterioration of marital quality (Filsinger & Thoma, 1988) and may be as important in determining marital satisfaction as are the actual behaviors the couple exchanges (Broderick & O'Leary, 1986). It is also clear that learning to show caring for your partner, even when you yourself are having a bad day, is a particularly important lesson for the depressed, discordant couple.

A third essential aspect of caring gestures is that their performance be recognized. It is necessary for the therapist to gain a good understanding of what gestures are being done, when, and by whom in order to monitor the impact of the intervention. It is also very important for the members of a depressed, discordant couple to learn to recognize caring gestures when they occur and to take the time to feel good that their spouse has done this for them. To this end, we typically use *self-monitoring* by the spouses, whereby each spouse records what caring gestures he/she performed. However, we have the spouses record their gestures in the same place, so that each spouse has the opportunity to be "informed" about what the other spouse is doing. Having individuals record their own behavior rather than that of their spouse further emphasizes individual responsibility for increasing positive interactions and helps to avoid the induction of negative attributions for the partner's increased positive behavior. Each spouse's having ongoing access to the other's self-monitoring records also helps train both spouses to notice that more positive things are happening and to feel good about the positive change in their marriage. Particularly in the case of the depressed, discordant couple, it should not be assumed that an increase in positive, caring behavior will automatically be noticed. Close monitoring of the success in implementing the caring-gestures assignment allows the therapist to identify potential problems as well as particularly effective behaviors. At the same time, it provides a natural forum for inquiring about each spouse's ability to notice and appreciate the partner's behavior. This naturally emphasizes increased positive tracking.

Finally, it is important that spouses be taught ways of reinforcing the caring behavior of their partner. It is not at all uncommon in depressed, discordant couples for the spouses to respond "blankly" to a partner's caring behavior. Sometimes they report feeling entitled to the gesture and so believe responding positively would be inappropriate, but often it will simply not have occurred to them that a response was called for.

We have found it necessary to be careful in introducing the concept of reinforcement to depressed, discordant couples. Many spouses will respond negatively to any idea that sounds like a suggestion that they "manipulate" or "work at influencing" or "reward" their partner for engaging in more desirable, caring behavior. In some cases this negative reaction appears to reflect a strong sense of entitlement to this behavior from the spouse (e.g., "He should do it without my needing to say anything"); in other cases it may reflect a desire to be "loved for myself" (e.g. "If I 'reward' him for doing these things they won't reflect his love for me"). While these reactions may, in some cases, reflect underlying dysfunctional beliefs about marriage, we have not found the opening stage of therapy to be a good time to work on modifying such beliefs. Thus, with depressed, discordant couples we present the idea of reinforcement under the general framework of "open communication with the spouse." We discuss with the couple the importance of letting their partner know that he/she is on track and doing well when performing caring items. This is presented as important information that allows the partner to select items that maximize positive impact. We then discuss ways for each spouse to honestly and forthrightly inform the other that a caring gesture has been noticed and its intent appreciated, as well as how to communicate the feelings it evoked. We also discuss ways to compliment the behavior directly, to show positive facial affect in response to the behavior, and to attend physically to the partner while making the comment. In each case, we introduce simple versions of communication guidelines that will be further refined later in therapy. We have found that this approach allows couples to dramatically increase their rate of mutual reinforcement while effectively sidestepping issues of entitlement and control. We build on these skills further when we work with couples to enhance self-esteem in the marriage.

Creating a good caring-gesture list may take one or more sessions. The exercise of having each spouse generate possible caring items for him/herself and for the partner is also an excellent introduction to objectification (Weiss, 1978) and rudimentary communication skills. We typically have the couple work together to create one master list of caring items that contains all the items generated by each partner individually as well as by the two of them together. We cut out the center of a normal $8\frac{1}{2}" \times 11"$ pad of paper and write the items generated on the last page of the pad. The "flaps" of the cut-out pad allow each spouse to monitor his/her own performance of caring items on a daily basis. Table 5-1 is an example of a possible caring-gesture list, including some idiosyncratic items.

It is particularly important that no particular item on the list ever be mandatory. All behaviors are to be exchanged freely and without coercion. This allows more items to be included, with fewer concerns about possible negative reactions. In fact, it can be pointed out that the larger the pool of items, the more options each spouse has. Sometimes couples will wonder if they can add items later. While this type of continuing creative involvement in the assignment should be encouraged, spouses should also be encouraged to bring the new items into the session before actually writing them on the list.

## Caring Days

Besides using the technique of increasing the frequency of small caring gestures, the therapist can also suggest a more time-consuming and more difficult (but potentially very effective) technique called caring days (Stuart, 1980) or love days (Weiss et al., 1973). As implied by the name, caring days are whole days (or afternoons or evenings) that are devoted to showing love and caring for one spouse by the other. Caring days are

TABLE 5-1. Sample Caring-Gesture List

| | |
|---|---|
| Go out for breakfast once a week | Tom will initiate sensual interactions |
| Jill will wear red lipstick/nailpolish | Jill will initiate sexual interactions |
| Jill will wear red lingerie | Express verbal affection to spouse |
| Go out for an evening's entertainment | Jill will talk louder |
| Go for a walk | Tom will buy Jill flowers |
| Go for a ride | Share feelings and thoughts with spouse |
| Have a drink together | Hold hands |
| Have a romantic dinner | Lie on sofa together |
| Give spouse a massage | Show physical affection to spouse in |
| Take a shower together |   private |
| Jill will be a good sport about Tom's | Show physical/verbal affection in front |
|   teasing |   of others |
| Jill will give Tom things to laugh about | Compliment spouse |
| Give spouse hug/kiss when I come | Hold hands with spouse while driving |
|   home | Jill will bake a pie |
| Write note to tell spouse that he/she is | Tom will tape Phil Donahue's show |
|   appreciated | Spouse will listen sympathetically |

designed and implemented totally by one partner for the benefit of the other. For example, a husband may arrange for a babysitter, purchase groceries, cook a favorite dinner for his wife, and take her to a movie. As with caring gestures, it is very important that the spouse try to choose activities that are favorites of the *partner*. Because they require more investment in terms of time and (usually) money, caring days also have a higher potential for failure than do caring gestures. Caring days should probably not be assigned until the therapist has a good idea about the capacities of the spouses in terms of imagination, motivation, and ability to "read" the partner's preferences. Thus they are probably not a good choice for an initial intervention with a depressed, discordant couple but may be used later in therapy if needed and appropriate.

## Companionship Activities

Therapeutic interventions aimed at increasing pleasant shared activities also directly address dyadic cohesion. Depressed, discordant couples typically function as married isolates, living separately under one roof. Thus we place a great deal of stress on increasing companionship and shared activities and routinely expect to do work with couples on increasing joint positive activities, such as dating, joint recreational activities, and activities with other couples. This can be surprisingly difficult. One couple declared that there were absolutely no activities they would both enjoy doing; they were simply too different. The therapist gently probed for activities they used to do together while they were dating and during the early, childless years of their marriage. It turned out that there were many activities that they used to engage in, but each assumed that the other would no longer be interested in such "childish" recreational things as going to baseball games, going bowling, or going camping. Simply because they had not done such things for years, they had begun to see them as "things we don't do." This couple was particularly successful at initiating and enjoying shared activities once they overcame their initial reluctance.

Once again, the therapist must be on guard for suggestions for joint activities that have a high likelihood of failure. If one partner sounds unenthusiastic, or if the activity depends on some outside circumstance (e.g., "If I can get half-price tickets, then we'll see a Broadway show"), the suggestion should be further examined, and, if appropriate, a backup activity should be identified. If a joint activity fails at this stage, each spouse can react by blaming and displaying punitive behavior toward the other. For example, a couple we saw attempted to go out for dinner together as a shared activity early in therapy. The husband neglected to make reservations at a particular restaurant his wife had mentioned she would like to try. When they got to the restaurant, they were turned away because of the lack of a reservation. The wife took this opportunity to focus on the "irresponsibility" and "insensitivity" of her husband rather than on the fact that he left work early and made a special effort to take her out. In turn, the husband saw his wife as "demanding" and "impossible" instead of seeing his role in the problem.

Since one of the purposes of the initial assignments aimed at increasing positive interactions is to create a positive emotional climate and give the couple a sense of hope and mastery, it is especially important to guard against unnecessary failure at this stage. One of the best ways to do this is for the therapist to be quite detailed when making homework assignments. Especially when first getting to know a couple, the therapist should make no assumptions about their abilities to carry out "simple" assignments. Thus, for the couple mentioned above whose dinner date was unsuccessful, the therapist might have prevented the failure by asking detailed questions about exactly how the date was to be carried out. Who is to decide the evening? Who is to decide the place? When will this decision be made? What might get in the way of enjoyment of the evening? Are there any actions that might be taken to minimize the likelihood of an unenjoyable evening? It is wise for the therapist to assign responsibility for various aspects of a task to one or the other partner, since "joint responsibility" frequently translates into "no one's responsibility." Thus the husband mentioned above could have been responsible for contacting a babysitter and getting off work early, while the wife could have been in charge of selecting a restaurant and making reservations. Decisions about who should have what task will vary with the inclinations of the particular couple and may be influenced by the therapist's view of what would be therapeutic for the structure of the relationship (this will be discussed in more detail in the next chapter). It is important to note that at this early stage of therapy, the therapist typically will not let the couple attempt to problem solve in order to arrive at an optimal division of labor. Rather, the therapist is likely to be very involved in helping determine who does what.

## Sexual Interaction

Sexual interactions can be shared positive events, of course, but it is imperative that the therapist carefully assess the status of sex in the couple's relationship before accepting sexual and sensual items as part of a caring-gesture list early in therapy. It is common for distressed couples to report some sexual problem (O'Leary & Arias, 1983), and loss of libido is a common symptom of the depressive syndrome. Thus sexual problems are likely to be particularly common in this population. If there are sexual problems in a relationship, it is taking a significant risk for a therapist to suggest incorporating sexual interactions into their shared positive time. It is entirely possible that sexual interaction may *not* be positive for one or both partners. If it appears that there are significant sexual problems, sex therapy procedures may be implemented along with other techniques later in therapy (Kaplan, 1974; LoPiccolo & LoPiccolo, 1978; Heiman, Lo-Piccolo, & LoPiccolo, 1976; Zilbergeld, 1978). The couple should be told that the sexual problems will be addressed. However, the purpose of the shared activities prescribed early in therapy is simply to initiate a warmer emotional environment so that the likelihood of success at improving the relationship (sexually as well as otherwise) will be enhanced later in the therapy process. Indeed, it is not inappropriate for the therapist to "ban" sexual activity early in therapy if it is very unpleasant for one spouse, with the understanding that it will be addressed later in therapy.

## Increasing Individual Activities

It is common for depressed spouses to state directly or indirectly that they expect all of their satisfaction to be derived from activities involving their partners or provisions supplied by their partners. This represents a significant barrier to achieving an optimal level of couple cohesion and also prevents the depressed spouse from adequately using his/her individual resources in combating the depression. In addition, it is a rare spouse who does not reflexively back away from increased cohesion and intimacy when faced with the specter of being responsible for all aspects of the depressed partner's satisfaction. Thus we commonly encourage the depressed spouse to pursue independent interests more actively at the same time that we are encouraging increased joint activities.

A situation we have encountered frequently is that of a depressed wife who has small children at home and, as a consequence, has ceased many individual activities she once found pleasurable or satisfying. Depressed wives in this situation can experience serious problems of fatigue, mental strain, and loneliness. In addition, the depressed wife may unrealistically believe that her husband can or should make up for this strain. Thus, in addition to their direct effect on stress, the isolation and strain of childcare can produce another focus of marital discord. In one case we saw, there was an immediate upswing in mood on the wife's part as soon as the couple agreed that she should begin using a babysitter one afternoon a week. During her free afternoon, she indulged herself in clothes shopping, watercolor painting, visiting friends, or even napping or bathing in her own house. For some couples, the availability or the cost of babysitting is prohibitive. In these cases, it is essential that some creativity be used in putting together an arrangement by which the primary caretaker (usually the mother) can get some relief. Typically, providing opportunities for a mother to engage in independent pleasant activities results in enhanced cohesion for the couple as well as direct positive mood induction for the mother.

## Increasing Self-Esteem Support

A second aspect of the marriage that is in need of rapid repair early in therapy is its function in self-esteem support. While caring behaviors and shared activities convey a sense of valuing the partner, they typically do so indirectly. In addition to these indirect ways of providing self-esteem support, it is possible to intervene to increase the rate of positive spouse references, or, more simply, positive communication and positive tracking (Jacobson & Margolin, 1979). "Positive communication," as we are using it here, is not as difficult and involved as the set of behaviors that are normally the focus of communication training. By positive communication, we mean verbalizations that communicate appreciation or acknowledgment of the other person's good qualities or behavior. Positive communication of this sort, like the caring behaviors discussed above, is *independent* of the partner's perceived reciprocity. One person can choose to give a compliment or say "thank you" without cooperation on the part of the other person. Because it is not dependent on partner change, positive communication has less potential for failure than more complicated interactions, such as problem solving or empathic listening. Additionally, as opposed to many other aspects of communication training, verbalizations regarding appreciation and acknowledgment are already within the response repertoire of most clients, although they may be underused. Therefore, positive communication can be introduced to couples early in therapy (cf. Jacobson & Margolin, 1979).

When we introduce positive communication to clients, we usually present the concept as "expressing what you normally take for granted." In other words, we attempt to get them to verbalize thanks for the many tasks that their partner does for them (e.g., "Honey, you always iron my shirts so nicely; I appreciate it"); to acknowledge desired change in their partner (e.g., "I noticed that you have been putting your dirty dishes in the sink this past week; thanks a lot"); to give compliments (e.g., "You really look nice in that jacket"); and to express positive beliefs and feelings about their partner (e.g., "One of the things I love about you is your smile; I love it when you smile like this").

For some couples, the low rate of positive communication is simply a matter of having habituated to the partner. With prompting from the therapist, such clients will have no problem in increasing the frequency of their acknowledgment and appreciation responses. However, for other couples there may be initial obstacles to implementing the therapist's suggestion to increase positive communication that may or may not have surfaced earlier in the discussion of acknowledging caring gestures. One frequently articulated objection to increased positive communication among the nondepressed husbands we have dealt with is, "She should already *know* that I appreciate her; we got married, didn't we?" Another common objection is the idea that positive change should not be acknowledged because the partner is now only doing what *should* have been done years before. For both of these beliefs, we usually present the clients with a rationale for compliance that sidesteps any issues of blame or control. For example, we may suggest to a wife, "If you want your husband to increase a given behavior, you must inform him that you *like* it. If he is trying to do things you would like, and if you say nothing, he is likely to assume he made a mistake and you didn't like it after all." At the same time, we highlight the importance of each spouse as a source of daily information for the other about what is going well. If they fail to provide each other with positive observations that are accurate, it becomes very easy for these positive observations to be lost altogether. When this happens, their views of themselves are more vulnerable to threats and more likely to become distorted in a negative direction. Thus we explain that being able to express positives, compliments, and appreciation is very important both for helping keep the relationship on the best course as well as providing a more accurate view of themselves and their relationship. In addition, we emphasize the importance of being able to communicate genuine appreciation in a sincere manner. It is only honest and genuine positive observations that provide any benefit to the relationship.

Specific examples of positive communication that a particular couple would probably have the opportunity to try out during the following week should be listed in session and practiced. The therapist can start out by asking the clients to give a compliment or verbalize appreciation to each other in session. Some clients will have no problems doing this. However, if the clients are reluctant to do this task, or if they are unsuccessful in verbalizing the positive statement in a truly positive manner, either because of the choice of words or because of concurrent nonverbal behavior (voice tone or posture), the therapist should model the desired response. The therapist can then have each spouse repeat the modeled behavior, with the therapist playing the role of the other spouse. Then the therapist can step out of the picture and have the clients give positive statements directly to each other. Not until this has been success-fully completed should the clients be sent home with the homework assignment of increasing their positive communication with each other.

Once positive communication as outlined above has been initiated, it is often appropriate and useful to focus attention on the recipient's response to the positive communications. Because the recipient's re-sponse to a positive statement can either reinforce or punish that state-ment, this process must also be clarified for clients at an early stage in therapy. The therapist can model a good response to a compliment (e.g., "Oh, I'm really glad you like the meal; thanks") as well as poor or punishing responses (e.g., "I never heard that out of you before," "You're just saying that," or a negative nonverbal response such as a disdainful stare).

Just as with caring gestures, it is important for the therapist to get a good idea of how much positive communication is going on at home. We often have clients monitor their positive communication on the same paper as the one they use to monitor caring gestures.

## Reducing or Eliminating Major Stressors: An Initial Focus on Negative Patterns

A distressed marital relationship is not only a poor source of marital support; it is frequently an active source of stress. Sometimes before therapy can begin the process of healing the relationship, it is necessary to address the ongoing patterns in the marriage that may be inflicting damage on the depressed as well as the nondepressed spouse. Clearly, it is difficult for old wounds to heal when fresh ones are being inflicted every day. Thus, when we discover salient, ongoing negative behavior, we pinpoint it as a target of immediate change. In a number of studies it has been shown that negative behavior has a stronger association with satis-faction levels than does positive behavior (e.g., Broderick & O'Leary, 1986). Thus a relatively low number of very negative interactions may have the effect of wiping out a greater number of positive interactions. In addition, destructive behavior that is severely distressing in its own right may occur. This is behavior that is so negative in itself as to become a focus of dissatisfaction, independent of the issue that elicited it. In particular, we have found that verbal and physical aggression, threats to terminate the relationship, derogating references, high levels of criticism and blame, or behaviors that unilaterally produce severe disruption of marital routine (such as not coming home at night or leaving the house after arguments) can be extremely destructive for both the marriage and the depressed spouse. If allowed to occur, they will completely stop or at least severely impede progress in therapy. We conceptualize these maladaptive behaviors as almost always being methods, albeit coercive methods, of dealing with problems in the relationship (Patterson & Reid, 1970). However, these methods themselves prevent any progress in dealing with the underlying problems. Therefore, we put great emphasis on eliminating these destructive behaviors as early in therapy as possible. When we do so, we emphasize to our clients that this early "suppression" of negative behaviors is not the eventual goal of marital therapy. We assure them that we will deal with problems in therapy, but in a much different way and in a context that allows for positive feelings to coexist with problem discussions. Thus partners are not asked to "make sacrifices" or "compromises" at this early stage in therapy. They are, however, asked to stop some forms of negative behavior that will prevent them from finding effective ways to deal with problems.

For most moderately discordant couples (Dyadic Adjustment Scale [DAS] scores between 50 and 97), the salient negative behaviors we make the focus of early directives are essentially voluntary and controllable given the context of a program of therapy aimed at resolving grievances in the near future. For some severely discordant couples (DAS scores between 10 and 50), it is our impression that the severely maladaptive behavior patterns that tend to preclude an initial positive focus sometimes may be less voluntary and controllable. For these couples, the therapist's directive to change, even coupled with a strong rationale and reassurance about addressing problems later in the course of therapy, may not be sufficiently potent to produce change. While there is little concrete evidence at present regarding this issue, our clinical impression is that severely discordant couples will often show repeated breakthroughs of the high-intensity disruptive interactions described above. For these couples, it may be necessary to alter the course of therapy to use structured individual interventions aimed at increasing each spouse's self-control of disruptive behavior before a dyadic focus can prove useful (cf. Jacobson & Margolin, 1979). Alternatively, it may sometimes be possible to effectively address these high-intensity negative interactions by using cognitive marital therapy techniques currently being developed (cf. Baucom & Epstein, 1990; Beach & Bauserman, 1990). A third alternative with these severely discordant couples is suggested by the observation that in some of these cases a lifting of the depressive episode will occur if the decision is made to divorce or separate. Thus it may be appropriate in some cases to focus on individual therapy for the depressed patient and support the process of disengaging from the relationship.

Below, each of the most common marital "stressors" is examined, along with helpful techniques that can be offered to couples. In addition, if a particular idiosyncratic behavior is found to be negative, threatening, and chronic, it should also be dealt with as a major stressor in the relationship.

## Denigrating, Criticizing, and Blaming Spousal References

Blaming and devaluing a partner through excessive criticism can be seen as a major and chronic stressor in marriage. We deal with this issue by giving explicit feedback about the detrimental effects of such behavior and explicitly directing spouses to stop engaging in name-calling and spousal put-downs. In addition, we commonly present a conceptualization of the criticism-evoking behavior that can help the critical spouse reattribute the reasons for it. When spouses come to see the destructive nature of spousal criticism and put-downs, and also come to a different understanding of the behavior they are criticizing, we find that most of them are able to substantially decrease this behavior.

If the other spouse is seen as a blameworthy person who has intentionally acted destructively toward the marriage, however, then anger and continued spousal put-downs may be expected (Fincham et al., 1987). In addition, clients typically do not entertain the notion that there may be other ways to look at the situation besides their own. They are convinced that theirs is the correct view of the situation and may have little insight into their own contribution to the problem situation. Indeed, the fundamental attributional bias (Ross, 1977) suggests that most people tend to attribute their own behavior to situational factors while attributing others' behavior to intrapersonal factors. Thus, when I scream at my spouse I simply am responding to my spouse's unacceptable behavior, but when my spouse screams at me, he/she is acting out his/her trait of being nasty. If the therapist can reattribute the cause of the problems from internal, stable, blameworthy attributes of the spouse (e.g., "He's totally inconsiderate, always has been") to situationally determined, changeable, nonblameworthy factors (e.g., "His behavior is a dysfunctional attempt to improve the marriage"), the intense blame and negative affect may be decreased, along with the problematic spousal denigration. Thus, if the attribution can be changed, it may be possible to get back on track in therapy.

We usually attempt to reattribute problems by portraying them as symmetrical, mutually caused interaction patterns (cf. Baucom & Epstein, 1990; Fincham, Bradbury, & Grych, 1990). Since this represents our understanding of the interaction dynamic for most maritally discordant couples, it typically presents little difficulty. For example, we might explain to a couple that "Ben's attempts to calm things down and save the marriage have taken the form of being nonresponsive in the face of Helen's screaming, while Helen's attempts to breathe life back into the marriage have taken the form of trying to force a response from Ben by screaming even louder. The more Ben is nonresponsive, the more Helen yells, and vice versa. Both of you are involved, but neither has negative intent, or negative motivation, or is being selfish. Both of you are doing your best to help resolve the problem you both see as being present in your relationship." When successful, this type of reconceptualization of the problem fits naturally into the ongoing process of therapy and can help decrease blame dramatically. In turn, the decrease in blame and changed understanding of the partner's behavior tends to increase the ability of the couple to work productively together in marital therapy.

Another approach to changing the couple's understanding of each other's behavior involves portraying the intense blame and anger that are driving the spousal criticism and put-downs as the result of "miscommunication" or "misunderstanding." In these cases, exploring the differing *meanings* attributed to certain behaviors by each spouse may lead to a beneficial cognitive change. For example, for several couples with whom we have worked, the wives viewed a lack of conversation and romantic actions as indicating a lack of intimacy and closeness. The husbands in these marriages saw the lack of conversation and presence of parallel activities (e.g., both partners reading, working on separate projects, or watching television) as indicating relaxation and comfort with the other person. The husbands viewed "small talk" and "artificial niceness" as indications of *lack* of intimacy. Simply pointing out the different meanings behind the same behaviors did not change the partners' differing preferences for type of interaction with their mates, but it did help diffuse the feelings of anger and rejection that accompanied the original understanding. The diffusion of negative feelings set the stage for less spousal criticism and name-calling and led ultimately to productive problem solving to change the interaction patterns in ways that would be acceptable to both partners.

Another method of reducing blame and spousal criticism, which is nearly always appropriate for couples containing a depressed member, is to give information regarding the nature of the syndrome of depression. Many people do not understand that lethargy, lack of concentration, sleep disturbance, self-focus, irritability, and loss of sexual appetite are common manifestations of depression. Any of these symptoms could easily become the focus of marital discord in the absence of appropriate information. Indeed, we have interviewed couples whose primary "marital" complaints consisted entirely of symptoms of depression (e.g., "She's irritable all the time and we haven't made love for months"). These couples are helped simply by the information that such behaviors are not necessarily intrinsic to the depressed person and will probably improve as the depression lifts. Such information can also do much to diffuse blame of the depressed individual, particularly when the symptoms being complained of are negative symptoms of depression (e.g., lack of energy, lack of desire, lack of interest in others or usual activities; cf. Hooley, Richters, Weintraub, & Neale, 1987). Thus, when dealing with the stressor of spousal denigration, we attempt to directly suppress the behavior, but we are also ready to work cognitively with the couple to explore the sources of their frustration, anger, and blame. When a spouse is helped to come to a new understanding of the partner's behavior, it often becomes possible for him/her to change the maladaptive pattern of criticism, blame, and denigration.

## Verbal and Physical Abuse

In a sample of newly married couples, 41% of the women and 33% of the men reported using physical violence in conflicts with their partners (O'Leary et al., 1989). The use of violent interactions in early marriage is common but is not always reported to be a problem. For couples who are distressed, however, verbally or physically abusive tactics may always be viewed as contributing to the couples' problems. With abusive couples, we attempt to give the abusive partners some specific techniques to limit their anger and stop an abusive escalation before it starts. At the same time, we emphasize that the issues from which the abusive situations emanate will be dealt with later in therapy. With a frequently physically abusive couple, we introduce time-out procedures in the first session. This takes priority over any other issue because of the destructiveness, both physical and movitational, of abusive incidents. Time-out procedures to prevent anger escalation and abusive incidents consist of each partner monitoring his/her own anger level and asking *calmly* to have time-out from the situation when he/she begins to get angry. The spouses then physically separate for as long as it takes them to become calm again. Once calm, they attempt to resume the discussion. If they become angry again, they call time-out again. The couple may agree to postpone discussion of the anger-producing topic until they see their therapist. There are several essential points regarding the implementation of time-out. First, each partner must try to *prevent* an angry escalation, which means they should err on the side of calling time-out too early rather than too late. Second, when one partner calls a time-out, it must be respected by the other partner, even if the other partner is not angry. One scenario thought to be common in prompting abusive incidents consists of one party attempting to leave the situation and the partner preventing this by pursuit or physical restraint. Accordingly, both partners must agree in session that they will respect the request for time-out when their partner makes it. Third, when couples physically separate, it is usually better for both of them to remain *within* their home, with the two spouses in separate rooms if possible, rather than for one partner to leave the home. Finally, they must attempt to discuss the issue after they have calmed down or else make a future appointment to do so. This last requirement is necessary to prevent one partner from using time-out to avoid necessary discussions.

The therapist should model how to call a time-out; it should be done calmly and nonprovocatively. For example, "I'm getting angry, let's have a time-out" rather than, "There you go again, making me crazy; I'm leaving." The therapist should have the partners role-play, asking for a time-out in session until they can do it appropriately. This should be continued until it is clear that it can be done appropriately. If a time-out is requested in an inappropriate or provocative manner, it can instigate the very behavior it is supposed to prevent.

If it appears that anger and abuse are not being controlled by the therapist's emphasis on the unacceptability of these behaviors and by the implementation of time-out, then it is likely that the couple could benefit from a more structured approach to anger control and elimination of abuse, such as the one detailed by Arias and O'Leary (1988). Regardless of the approach used, when physical abuse is ongoing, it must be the primary focus of therapy.

## Threats to Leave the Relationships

Many couples may come for marital therapy after already beginning to contemplate divorce. Sometimes these couples are caught in a pattern of threatening to leave whenever an argument or other negative experience occurs. This pattern is an impediment to the occurrence of real progress. Even in the most successful course of marital therapy, there will be bad days and even bad weeks. If the couple is in the habit of threatening to end the relationship, a bad day can become the final straw rather than an opportunity to learn from some mistakes. We take the position that it is understandable to have ambivalence about continuing a relationship in which things have been rocky. In addition, depression in oneself or one's partner tends to bias individuals toward being more pessimistic about everything. Thus occasional thoughts of divorce are natural. We encourage couples to see thoughts of divorce as disturbing intrusions with little information value (other than confirming that they are depressed and maritally discordant). We also note that in order to be successful in marital therapy, it is necessary to use therapy as an opportunity to learn about marriage and making marriage work. A partner who learns how to "make marriage satisfying" has gained a great deal that will be helpful in many areas of life regardless of whether the marriage survives. However, we are quick to remind couples of the evidence that they care about each other and are deeply invested in each other's lives and to suggest that their threats of divorce reflect only temporary feelings, not their deeper and more compelling desires to make things work. In addition, we stress that although they may still have occasional thoughts regarding leaving, it is not helpful to verbalize these thoughts to the spouse, since these thoughts occur in an inconsistent, vacillating pattern rather than representing a final decision. Thus impulsively sharing fleeting thoughts of divorce with the spouse actually decreases understanding and accuracy rather than clarifying their feelings about the relationship.

Some individuals who are very low in commitment to their marriage or very discordant continue to threaten their spouses with the end of the relationship in an inconsistent, vacillating manner. Such behavior may be dealt with in an individual session in which the therapist can be confrontational with the client, pointing out that this behavior is in effect sabotaging the therapy. The therapist can further probe to discover whether the individual has actually resolved to end the relationship and is doing so in a passive rather than direct manner. If the client has in fact decided to leave, the therapist can offer to help him/her inform the other spouse.

## Disruption of Scripted Marital Behavior

Sometimes the spouse of a depressed patient will show virtually no interaction with the depressed individual. In our own experience, this has typically occurred when the husband has work-related "obligations" that keep him from such activities as eating dinner with the wife or family, spending time at home in the evening, talking with his wife about daily occurrences, or taking part in special family occasions or events. This pattern of behavior appears to function as a major stressor for the depressed wife, as well as undermining any attempt to increase cohesion. While this type of behavior will sometimes be associated with undisclosed extramarital sex, it also appears to result from workaholic behavior patterns or severe job stress. The effect of this type of behavior is to disrupt normal patterns of marital interaction and leave a void of scripted behavior for the couple. The result is a pattern that generates considerable depressive symptomatology for the depressed partner.

When such a pattern exists, the husband will often claim to be unable to attend marital therapy. The therapist may then be forced to do individual therapy, even though marital discord appears relevant to the depression. If the husband is willing to participate, the establishment of routines and patterns in the couple's daily interaction must take some priority in therapy. We have found it useful to establish some set times when the couple will make contact every day and to set times when prolonged interaction will be possible. Mealtimes are often useful in this regard, but alternatives may include some combination of phone calls, notes, evening activities, going to bed at the same time, joint involvement in church or other social activities, or meeting during the day. Only after there is some predictability and reasonable frequency to the contact between the spouses is it possible to work on making that contact more positive.

## Idiosyncratic Major Marital Stressors

Many types of behavior and interaction can take on special meaning for a particular couple. When this special shared meaning is extreme and negative, it is necessary for the therapist to intervene as would be done regarding any other major marital stressor. Worthy of special mention is one situation we have seen often enough to consider including it among the common major marital stressors. This is the situation of the depressed, discordant wife being left alone with her small children, rarely getting out and unable to share emotionally with her husband. We discussed strategies for dealing with this situation earlier. However, here we would emphasize that there is data suggesting a link between small children at home and depression (Brown & Harris, 1978). In our clinical work we have found that this situation can function as a stressor, preventing both symptomatic improvement and marital improvement for the depressed, discordant mother unless it is addressed directly. Another idiosyncratic marital stressor we have seen involves one partner's using alcohol or other substances in a manner that the other partner finds very objectionable. For example, in one case a wife who had grown up with an alcoholic father found any alcohol consumption by her husband to be extremely distressing. In other cases, the substance use may be abusive and may create financial or other hardship. Likewise, we have seen cases in which interactions with in-laws were a major source of stress, with one spouse's involvement with his/her family of origin precipitating recurring feelings of abandonment and rejection in the other. In some cases particular behaviors may carry unusual stress because of their prior association with acts of infidelity or unreliability. *Any* behavior that engenders high levels of recurrent stress is a candidate for change early in therapy.

## Process Issues in the Initial Phase of Therapy

### The Role of the Therapist

We will now present some goals and issues concerning the therapist's role and function that are independent of the social support model but that are important for engaging depressed, discordant couples in the therapy process.

#### SOCIALIZATION INTO THERAPY

The initial phase of therapy has another purpose apart from the particular behavior changes sought. The clients are also learning what is expected of them in the therapy situation. Even if clients have been in therapy before, they must learn the expectations of this therapist and this particular program of therapy. The interventions employed early in therapy, therefore, are also important with regard to what they are teaching the client couple about therapy. To the extent that they are teaching "metalessons" that will be useful in later phases of therapy, early interventions are doubly useful to the therapist. The early intervention techniques discussed above have in common that they teach several important lessons about the general therapy process.

First, they teach clients about homework. The process of deciding on appropriate homework, explaining it to the clients, and evaluating their degree of success with last week's assignment takes up much of the session time and is essential to improvement. We have found that compliance is indeed related to clinical improvement (Sandeen et al., 1987). Early success with homework emphasizes its usefulness to the clients, who may resist it at first if it is not part of their view of what therapy should be.

Individual responsibility for one's own behavior is another important lesson that emerges from doing homework. Each individual in the couple is responsible to the therapist for his/her homework assignment. There is no such thing as "joint responsibility," because with joint responsibility comes diffusion of responsibility and decreased motivation to act. Therefore, even in joint tasks, each individual is responsible for doing his/her part, *even if* the other spouse is uncooperative. Early assignments, such as caring gestures, underscore the responsibility of each person for his/her own behavior, independent of the spouse's behavior.

A third lesson that the early interventions teach about therapy is that it is action oriented. There is certainly "talking therapy" during the therapy hour, but a plan for action is decided on during that hour and is to be carried out before the next session. The therapist tries to model a problem-solving approach throughout therapy and in later stages actively teaches problem solving as a couple skill (see Chapter 6). Thus clients learn that they will identify problems, discuss alternatives, choose an alternative to carry out, try out the new alternative, and evaluate its degree of success (D'Zurilla & Golfried, 1971). This is a different orientation toward personal problems from the one many clients bring to therapy. This action-oriented approach, however, must take into account the fact that many depressed individuals feel immobilized by their depression. Early behavior-change assignments must be geared toward the depressed client's level of functioning in order to maximize the chance for successful completion of the assignment.

Yet another lesson clients learn very early on is that the therapist does not take sides in the marital dispute. The therapy hour is a time when spouses can be sure they will not be attacked by their partner or be allowed to attack. In addition, the therapist is on both their individual sides as well as on the side of the relationship. Thus the therapist's attitude conveys a strong sense of dual alliance and the expectation that win–win solutions are possible.

## THERAPIST-INDUCED EXPECTATIONS FOR IMPROVEMENT

The therapist, by virtue of his/her expert role, has the ability to give information that will be received as credible by clients. We try to turn the potential "placebo" effect of this situation to the client's advantage by expressing both implicit and explicit expectations for improvement. Thus early in therapy the therapist lays the groundwork for change by defining the clients' problems and goals in as specific a manner as possible. Implicitly, this process communicates to the clients that change is expected. Explicitly, we frequently give a short speech on the research background of the cognitive-behavioral marital therapy approach, emphasizing that many couples are helped to be more maritally satisfied within a relatively brief therapy process. In order to maintain credibility, it is important to remain "professional" and not become a salesperson for the therapy. For example, clients should not be "guaranteed" success, and other forms of therapy should not be denigrated as inferior in comparison to the cognitive-behavioral marital therapy orientation. Indeed, we have found it useful to tell couples of the many empirically supported, effective treatments for depression that are now available. We tell them that this approach can help them, and even if it does not, there are other approaches that might; that is, this approach has been determined to be a good one for them, but it is by no means their only hope for improvement. We have every expectation that we will work together successfully to relieve their depression and improve their marriage. In addition, we explain that we are working with the natural healing process, since most depressions tend to lift over time even in the absence of treatment. Anything that tends to increase the couple's expectation that they will experience positive change is potentially useful during the opening stage of therapy.

A second way in which the therapist can influence expectation of change is by working actively to foster the perception that change is occurring. Couples with a depressed member often focus on another problem as soon as one problem has seen improvement, creating the illusion that no change is occurring. In such instances, the therapist must work to help the clients perceive how far they have come since the beginning of therapy. The therapist can help clients remain aware of change to which they have habituated with such comments as, "Fran, it sounds like you felt dissatisfied with Tony's involvement with the children this week. Was he more involved with them this week than he was a month ago?" Depressed spouses may also show a tendency to discount positive achievements while inflating negative occurrences, making it even more important for the therapist working with depressed, maritally discordant couples to facilitate an accurate recognition that change is taking place.

## Common Early Problems
## That Can Sidetrack Therapy

Although each couple brings their own unique history and concerns to therapy, there are some issues that seem to come up frequently in the early stages of marital therapy with depressed spouses.

### THE "BIG ISSUE"

Although we recommend trying to increase hedonically positive events early in therapy, this strategy may not work for all couples. For some, the "big issue" or overwhelming concern with which they came into therapy feels too pressing to allow them to focus on increasing positive events. "Big issues" can include such topics as childbearing, whether or not to move, and prior affairs. We initially attempt to persuade clients to work on caring gestures and other changes before attempting larger issues. However, we occasionally fail to be sufficiently convincing. Rather than prescribing caring gestures or other positive behaviors only to have the assignment fail or be avoided by a spouse who is not ready to be constructive, we accede to the clients' wishes and deal with the "big issue." However, we make it clear that although we might be able to help them resolve this troublesome issue in the short term, the solution is likely to be temporary and patchwork. We explain that it will almost certainly be necessary to return to the issue again at a later point in therapy when they are more ready to resolve it. We might help the couple understand each other's perspectives on a specific problematic area, we might supply alternatives to try out, but we would not attempt to teach problem solving or communication skills in any formalized manner. In other words, any early intervention other than increasing positive interactions should be highly controlled by the therapist and should have as its immediate goal problem resolution rather than skill building. In this regard, dealing with the "big issue" for couples is rather like removing major but idiosyncratic stressors. It needs to be done so therapy can progress normally.

## PERCEIVED ARTIFICIALITY OF ASSIGNMENTS

Many couples have difficulty with the behavioral marital therapy model because it assumes a different relationship between feelings and behavior than does the typical layperson's view. Most people believe that action should come spontaneously from feelings. This view implies that if the positive feelings are not there, one cannot behave in a warm and giving manner. It also implies that feelings must change before action can change. Thus people who share this view may initially look askance at typical early assignments such as those outlined in this chapter. Assignments to "do nice things" for one another may be seen as artificial and useless if the clients believe that feelings must change before behavior can change.

In dealing with this issue, probably the most important thing the therapist can do is inquire about the clients' view of the therapy model and the homework assignments and openly acknowledge the reasonableness of their feelings. Clients usually are somewhat hesitant to bring up their opinions about what is done and said in therapy unless they are explicitly asked, but if their negative feelings about assignments are not directly dealt with, the likelihood is high that the homework will fail. Thus the first step is to acknowledge and validate the view of change that the clients bring to therapy.

The second step is to persuasively introduce another view, one consistent with behavioral marital therapy. To this end, we present the view that behavior and feelings are mutually determined. Positive behavior on the part of one's spouse leads to positive feelings and positive behavior toward oneself, leading to more positive feelings and behavior from the spouse, and so forth. Therefore, although there may be some feeling of artificiality at first, a natural cycle can be instigated, producing good feelings once the behavior becomes more positive. Most couples seem to accept this explanation at first, and if they have success in the first few assignments, they are sold on the model. In addition, as discussed earlier, we make a strong case that positive motives and inclinations are present in the couple and are being blocked or not expressed. Thus doing positive things together at times when they do not "feel like it" is not phony; it is a genuine expression of the same motives that brought them in for marital therapy.

## INTERFERENCE OF DEPRESSIVE SYMPTOMATOLOGY

Using marital therapy, we have successfully treated people who met DSM-III diagnostic criteria for major depressive episode (American Psychiatric Association, 1980) and who had initial Beck Depression Inventory scores in the 30s and 40s. Therefore, the presence of moderate to severe depression is not in itself a clear contraindication for marital therapy. However, if the depression is severe enough that the depressed individual is unlikely to successfully perform the caring gestures or positive communication assignments described in this chapter, marital therapy as presented here cannot take place. Whether marital therapy can be used successfully with a given couple can be gauged by the amount of time during the therapy hour spent on each of the two members of the couple. If the depressed member is requiring significantly more than half of the therapist's time, and especially if the therapist finds him/herself talking mainly about individual rather than couple issues, it may be necessary to discard the marital model, at least temporarily. If a depressed individual initially unable to participate effectively in marital therapy can be seen individually for a course of cognitive therapy or interpersonal psychotherapy, or is given antidepressant medication with some initial beneficial effect, marital therapy may then resume with greater positive effect.

DEALING WITH FAILURE

A large part of the strategy and technique of the initial phase of therapy is focused on preventing failure experiences and encouraging success experiences. As mentioned earlier, this is done in order to build positive expectations about therapy and to disrupt negative cognitions the clients may have regarding their own or their spouse's ability to change (Eidelson & Epstein, 1982). Nonetheless, early failures in carrying out assignments may occur. The therapist's reactions to the failure will be an important factor in whether the clients can overcome their rocky start or whether they will fail in the therapeutic endeavor. This is an especially important point when dealing with the depressed client. How can the therapist prevent failure from escalating? (1) The therapist can help the couple before the occurrence of a failure experience by exploring the possibility of failure. When we give assignments, we explore the possible reasons that an assignment might not work as planned. (2) The therapist can help the couple after the fact by turning failure into success. Often, the therapist can help the client learn something from a "failed" homework experience, and homework assignments should be designed with this in mind. Thus, whenever the therapist can aid a couple in understanding why an assignment was a failure, the couple should be praised for learning something important, and a new assignment taking into account the new information should be given. For example, if the couple was assigned to do a positive joint activity and it turned out to be unpleasant because one partner did not like the activity and had not previously said so, the couple should be praised for discovering this valuable information about one partner's preferences (as well as discovering the importance of honest assertion), and a joint activity that they both really would like to do should be selected and assigned as homework for that week.

## Case Example: John and Marie

John and Marie were a couple in their late 50s who had been married for 25 years. It was the second marriage for both. Both John and Marie were depressed when they entered therapy (Beck Depression Inventory scores of 28 and 25, respectively), although only Marie was diagnostically evaluated and satisfied DSM-III criteria for a diagnosis of major depressive episode (American Psychiatric Association, 1980). The main complaints with which they entered therapy were lack of intimacy and lack of sexual interaction. Assessment showed that John had an extremely physically demanding job, and his typical evening consisted of coming home, having dinner, and falling asleep at about 9:00 P.M. in front of the television. Marie had recently had a heart attack, which prevented her from returning to her job (she had worked throughout their marriage). Marie was spending all her time at home, seeing no one except John. She was not engaged in any significant enjoyable activities. Although the couple had friends, they had not seen them regularly for years. Both John and Marie agreed that they had problems with procrastination regarding chores and projects around the house, as well as in regard to potentially entertaining activities. They felt they were living separate, boring existences. Marie especially felt that John did not care about her due to his lack of affection and sexual interest in her. The couple shared interest and concern regarding their three grown children and their grandchildren. Their communication difficulties stemmed primarily from a paucity of communication on John's part; Marie was quite articulate and a good communicator but had given up due to John's scant interest in talking, which worsened with his depression. Marie's depressive symptoms consisted of dysphoric mood accompanied by daily crying spells; lack of concentration and motivation; and hopelessness about the future of the marriage. John's primary depressive symptoms were lack of motivation, fatigue, and irritability.

Overall, John and Marie displayed many of the deficits in hedonically positive activities that we have discussed throughout this chapter, and these deficits appeared to be important in maintaining marital discord and depression for both of them. For that reason, their course of therapy was particularly focused on increasing positive events. Following is a summary of the content of therapy during the early stages for John and Marie. Note that a detailed intake interview, focused on information gathering, had already occurred prior to session 1.

## Session 1

During the first session, much time was spent on identifying which of their problems were symptoms of depression and giving information regarding the nature of depression. John and Marie were happy to hear that their irritability, lack of motivation, and hopelessness about the future were symptoms tied to their depressions and would likely lift once their depressions lifted. Connections were also made between the number and quality of hedonically positive activities performed during this depressed phase in their lives, as compared to other times in their lives when they were not depressed. This was done by eliciting a history of the marriage, focusing especially on good periods and what was going on during those periods. In this way, John and Marie could see the relationship between their actions (e.g., seeing friends, going to movies together, pursuing hobbies) and their emotional states. Homework consisted of developing lists of caring gestures for themselves (i.e., what they would like their spouse to do for them).

## Session 2

John and Marie appeared at session 2 in somewhat better moods than they had displayed during session 1. They attributed this change to understanding that they might have some control over their depressions through their actions. They had done part of their homework but had not developed very complete lists. Most of the session was spent in generating items for the caring-gesture lists that fit the criteria desired: small, inexpensive, and within the repertoire of the other spouse. Homework consisted of giving them the caring-gesture lists and asking them to perform one or two caring gestures per day for the other person.

## Session 3

Session 3 started out poorly because John had not complied with the assignment, whereas Marie had. Marie felt very depressed because she perceived John's behavior as an indication of a lack of caring on his part. The therapist spent a large part of the session validating Marie's feelings, helping John articulate the reasons for his noncompliance to Marie, and helping Marie understand the positive feelings John had for her. John's reasons for not completing the homework had more to do with his own depression than with any negative feelings about Marie. In particular, his hopelessness and extreme lethargy had led him to procrastinate rather than complete the homework assignment. The therapist suggested a "5-minute plan" for dealing with depression-induced procrastination for both John and Marie. The suggestion was to do the thing about which they found themselves procrastinating for "just 5 minutes." If at the end of that time the person felt like stopping, he/she should stop. The therapist explained that getting started is often the hardest part of a task for someone who is depressed. Thus the failure to complete the homework was reinterpreted as a valuable learning experience both in terms of better understanding each other and of identifying the obstacles that needed to be addressed in marital therapy.

Perfectionism in completing marital therapy homework assignments was discouraged; doing any part of the homework assignment was to be considered a success. John and Marie were given an assignment to do at least two "5-minute plans" apiece during the next week. They were also assigned continued work on the caring gestures.


## Session 4

John and Marie came into the session beaming. They had tried the "5-minute plan" and found it very helpful in breaking the cycle of lethargy and depression that was interfering with the completion of marital therapy homework assignments (and other activities). John had been much more successful in performing caring gestures for Marie, although Marie had still done more for him than he for her. Part of the session was spent emphasizing the connection between their changed behavior and their changed mood. The remainder of the session was spent discussing individual activities they could engage themselves in (other than watching television) and generating joint activities that would be pleasurable. Since sex was a long-standing problem with this couple, it was explicitly banned by the therapist at this stage, but the couple was told that issues involving sex would be addressed directly later in therapy. The homework assignment consisted of doing one positive joint activity (which was decided on in detail during the session) and continuing with caring gestures.


## Session 5

John and Marie were both feeling very good and successful due to their experiences with the homework activities of the previous week. They had traveled to their married daughter's home in a neighboring state for the weekend, something they had not done for several months, and had enjoyed themselves. Again, the connection between their action and their mood and feeling about the marriage was emphasized by the therapist. However, Marie had still performed more caring gestures for John than he had for her. This was seen as a problem by both of them. The therapist intervened, suggesting that John needed to learn to take more responsibility for the state of the marriage and that Marie therefore needed to relax her responsibility. Thus the therapist suggested that John take all the responsibility in the next week for planning their joint activity and for performing caring gestures. Marie would only continue with "inconspicuous" displays of caring. Both were receptive to this homework assignment, since they acknowledged that it addressed a long-standing problem of unequal contributions to the marriage.

# 6

## Restructuring the Relationship: Themes and Techniques of Midtherapy

The techniques described in Chapter 5 were designed to produce an elevation of mood for the depressed patient, instill a sense that change is possible for both spouses, and set the stage for the harder work of restructuring the relationship. Specifically, the early techniques centered around improving marital support by: (1) increasing companionship and dyadic cohesion; (2) increasing spousal self-esteem support; and (3) eliminating salient marital stressors. While the positive change strategies presented in Chapter 5 are useful with most discordant, depressed couples, the middle phase of therapy needs to be tailored to the needs of the particular couple. Recent evidence suggests that a more flexible, individually tailored approach to marital therapy is well received by clients and may enhance maintenance of gains made in therapy (Jacobson, Schmaling, Holtzworth-Munroe, et al., 1989).

After the first phase of therapy is complete, it is likely that the couple will be showing observable signs of change. There may have been some initial lifting of the depression, and the therapist is likely to notice a general softening of spouse's attitudes toward each other. As can be seen in Figure 6-1, husbands' perceptions of their wives' symptoms rapidly become more accurate in the earliest stages of marital therapy. While their wives' symptoms are already beginning to decrease, husbands' perceptions of their wives' symptoms increase until both reports are at the same level. We have had the clinical impression that this coincides with wives' feeling "heard" for the first time by their partners. These early changes in the relationship also appear to mobilize the hope that perhaps the marriage could be different and more satisfying. Thus, when the

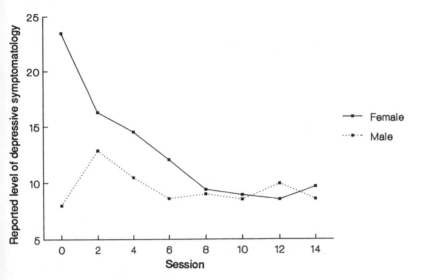

FIGURE 6-1. Wives' level of depressive symptomatology, reported by husbands and wives.

initial stage of therapy goes well, it sets the stage for the more difficult challenges that lie ahead.

If the first phase of therapy has gone well, the couple will have already shown an enhancement of cohesion and self-esteem support. Simultaneously, stressors associated with spousal denigration, concern over a partner's leaving the relationship, and ongoing disruption of scripted marital behavior will have subsided to a large extent. Although these areas typically continue to require some work, they need less intense, ongoing therapist attention. Thus the therapist can begin to attend to other relevant relationship areas, such as (1) increasing acceptance of emotional expression; (2) increasing the frequency and breadth of intimate exchanges; (3) enhancing perceived and actual coping assistance; (4) enhancing the perception of spousal dependability; (5) continuing to decrease sources of stress within the relationship; and (6) working on special problem areas of the couple. Problems in each of the areas can be glossed over by spouses in the first flush of successful marital change. However, if they are not dealt with during the course of therapy, the marital discord model would predict rapid relapse of marital discord and/or depressive symptomatology following termination.

Unfortunately, our clinical experience suggests that encouraging the couple to refocus on more problematic areas of the relationship will commonly result in a temporary increase in felt marital dissatisfaction.

As can be seen in Figure 6-2, there is usually a rapid response to the reduction of marital stressors and the focus on enhancing marital cohesion and self-esteem support. However, there is a reliable dip in reported satisfaction between sessions 4 and 6, as the couple begins to focus more on problem areas. We have found it useful to predict this temporary reaction and to interpret it as a normal part of the therapy process. This approach seems to help couples see their fluctuating marital satisfaction in context and prevents catastrophizing.

## Increasing Acceptance of Emotional Expression

Nearly all of our depressed, discordant couples receive communication training in one form or another aimed at increasing their ability to accept and listen to their partners. It is common for maritally discordant and depressed spouses to fail to listen to each other in a caring and attentive manner. Nondepressed husbands report that their wives' complaining or whining is aversive and that it has led to avoidance of problem discussion on their part. Depressed wives report that whenever they begin to discuss their feelings they find their husbands "tuning them out." The nondepressed husband also tends to see problem expression and complaining by the depressed wife as a sign of disaffiliation or rejection of the relationship, while she may see this behavior as a means of drawing closer (cf. Guthrie, 1988, cited in Weiss & Heyman, 1990). Thus misunderstanding and misperception can compound an already poor exchange of information.

The husbands in our depressed couples have often offered a minimal response or no response to their wives' complaints, as if they believed their lack of response would make the complaining go away. However, such nonresponse has only served to further aggravate their already deteriorated marital situation (Gottman & Krokoff, 1989). On the other hand, depressed wives have often been no better at listening to their husbands than their husbands were at listening to them. Commonly, when a husband would begin to discuss his view of a marital issue, the depressed wife would cut him off or immediately begin to vent emotions in response. This emotional venting would serve to powerfully inhibit further discussion on the husband's part, thereby feeding into his pattern of nonresponsiveness and further fueling the vicious cycle of negative exchange and withdrawal. Conversely, in some couples the partner of the depressed person would feel compelled to "cheer up" the depressed individual by giving suggestions about how he/she could feel better and downplaying the seriousness of the complaints voiced (cf. Stephens, Hokanson, & Welker, 1987). Usually, this would lead the depressed

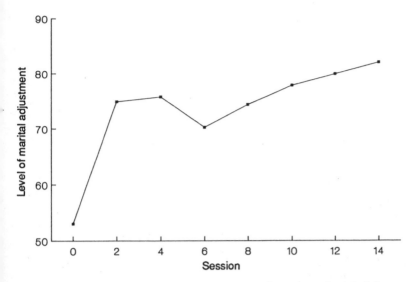

**FIGURE 6-2.** Wives' level of marital adjustment over the course of marital therapy for depression.

person to feel misunderstood, angry, and more depressed. Although the fear of the nondepressed spouse is that simply listening to the depressed partner and responding with empathy will increase the depression ("It will only encourage her"), we have found the opposite to be true. When the depressed wife feels that her partner is truly listening to her feelings and problems, she feels more hopeful and feels closer to him (cf. Guthrie, 1988). Accordingly, for both of these patterns, empathic listening training is potentially an effective antidote, one that both spouses need if acceptance of emotional expression is to be available within the context of the dyad. In addition, good listening skills will often further increase the level of cohesion in the dyad, allowing for increased self-esteem support, increased perceived availability of spousal support, enhanced couple problem solving, and the development of greater intimacy. Thus therapists often can initiate a number of beneficial processes by increasing empathic listening early in the middle stage of therapy.

## Empathic Listening: Course of Training

Usually we begin a communication training session by giving some information in a didactic manner. However, we try to keep this part of the training direct and brief, because we are interested primarily in developing a performance skill, not conceptual knowledge. We have found that improved performance stems from opportunities for the spouses to interact in the context of therapist structure and feedback rather than from didactic teaching methods used in isolation. In addition, we have found that our depressed, discordant couples have a particularly short attention span for the didactic component of marital intervention. Accordingly, we might begin a session on listener skills by saying something relatively simple such as,

> Tonight we're going to focus on listener skills. These are the skills that the person receiving the message can use in order to fully understand what is being said to them. This is *one* way of showing your partner that you are paying attention and care about what they have to say. But you will eventually change what we tell you and elaborate it so that it fits your "style." What is important is taking the time and effort to really listen and understand each other. The four listener skills we will focus on are: summarizing, reflecting, validating, and question asking [cf. Gottman, Notarius, Gonso, & Markman, 1976]. Let's get started with the first skill, summarizing. The point of summarizing is to break the cycle of each partner's saying their own message without responding to the message of the other person. By summarizing what you heard the other person say, you help your communication in two ways. First, you make certain you heard correctly what the other person is trying to say. If your summary is inaccurate, your partner has an opportunity to correct you. Second, you can show your partner that you value their message enough to really focus on it and listen rather than just going ahead with your own message. Now I'm going to give you some examples of summary statements and then you can try it yourselves.

It usually makes sense to introduce summarizing skills by first focusing on developing skills at the level of primary empathy (Egan, 1986). This type of summarizing is very content oriented. Only as this skill is mastered are more inferential, secondary-level empathic statements encouraged. As each spouse begins to practice listening skills, we have found it most effective to focus on one or two relatively salient issues at any given point. Typically, this is as much as clients can handle, and focusing on the most salient issues allows the clients to perceive more easily that they are changing and making progress.

As implied above, we move quickly from a didactic phase to a practice phase; first the therapist models the desired skills for the clients, and then the clients practice the skills with feedback from the therapist. It is usually helpful for the therapist to model the skills with one partner while role playing the husband or wife, then move to role playing with the other partner. Thus the wife might talk about a real problem she had with her husband during the past week while the therapist role plays the husband, using the skill of summarizing. Then the husband might talk about a problem he had during the past week while the role-playing therapist demonstrates summarizing. The clients themselves then practice summarizing, with the therapist again role playing the spouse. The therapist will stop and give feedback to the client who is practicing the skill, having him/her repeat the summarization until each has done it satisfactorily.

Giving feedback to a depressed individual must be done with special care. It must be remembered that the depressed person will tend to interpret feedback in a personal and global manner, perhaps concluding that "I can't do anything right; even my therapist says so." The therapist should try to find a positive aspect of the person's performance to comment on along with a negative aspect. Thus the therapist might say something like, "Susan, I liked how you kept your voice calm. That was good. But you didn't really summarize my statement. Instead you responded with your own statement. Let's try it again. Keep your nice calm voice and try to focus on summarizing what I say." Only after the clients have observed the therapist demonstrating the skill, and after they have successfully tried it with the therapist role playing the partner, are they encouraged to try it with each other. By starting communication training by using the therapist first as a model and then as a surrogate partner, we decrease the likelihood of unsuccessful experiences with the spouse, which can lead to a sense of futility and hopelessness. After successful in-session training in a particular skill, we assign homework to the couple in which they practice the skill for 5–15 minutes at home before the next session. We always attempt to have the couple tape-record these practice sessions. If at all possible, we encourage the couple to buy an inexpensive tape-recorder for this purpose. We strongly encourage tape-recording of home practice sessons because it enables us to critique the homework session during the next therapy hour and allows even a "disaster" to become a positive learning experience through the pinpointing of problem areas. If the homework session is not tape-recorded, then it becomes difficult to re-create either how it went wrong or what each person did that was helpful.

It is important to focus on the *skills* being taught in communication training. Clients typically will respond to the *content* of the communication in an emotional and overlearned manner. For example, when the therapist is attempting to teach the skill of summarization, the client who is speaking may bring up a "hot" topic. It will be extremely difficult to get the partner to simply respond with a summary statement to a topic that is laden with emotional baggage. If the response is not a successful attempt at calm summarization, the couple will begin their typical, unproductive sequence of interactions. It is essential that the therapist be very direct in stopping this sequence and redirecting the couple to the task of learning the skill at hand. Without firm direction at this stage, couples can become quite discouraged. Allowing discordant, depressed couples to argue in a nonconstructive manner for more than a brief period of time has such a negative effect on the therapeutic process with depressed patients that we do not usually allow negative interactions to continue in session for more than a few exchanges, even for assessment purposes.

Typically, we proceed through an informal hierarchy of problem topics over the course of several sessions, saving more difficult or "hotter" topics for later in therapy, when the couple is better equipped to deal with them constructively. Thus, if a couple has one or two "big issues" with which they have struggled unsuccessfully for a long time, we would ask them to put those issues on "the back burner" during the early training phases and use less emotionally charged topics to teach the skills. Since this is difficult for many clients to accept, we have found it helpful to give an actual estimate of a time when the problem issue will be approached. For example, if a couple is in their eighth session and is doing fairly well with learning communication skills using less important topics, the therapist may say, "I think we are almost ready to start on the topic of whether Jane should go back to school. Let's make our target date for this in 3 weeks from tonight, on the 25th. What do you think?"

## Empathic Listening Skills and Behavior

We usually focus on the four listener skills mentioned earlier—summarizing, reflecting, validating, and question asking—as well as commenting on nonverbal and attitudinal aspects of the listening process. However, the relative emphasis given to each depends on the clients' problem areas and ability to learn. Some clients have great difficulty understanding the concept of validation and never really succeed in doing it. However, if they can simply learn to summarize the partner's point of view in a calm manner rather than responding with angry criticism, they have learned a significant skill. Likewise, for some clients simply learning to face their partner directly with an open posture and not rush in too quickly with a reaction represents a significant advance. Thus the level of attainment that represents success in learning empathic listening skills depends on the needs and capacities of the particular couple involved in therapy. To continue to work on a particular skill for too long without making significant progress will often be worse for the process of therapy than accepting and working around residual areas of communication difficulty. Below we discuss several of the most common areas in which couples have difficulty and the skills that are taught to help remedy problems in each area.

## NONVERBAL BEHAVIOR

As alluded to above, nonverbal aspects of the interaction between spouses are very consequential in determining the impact of listening. A receptive and encouraging listening style does not come spontaneously for most discordant, depressed couples. The best nonverbal communication is a calm, relaxed posture: an open stance, with eye contact, perhaps leaning forward, and nodding appropriately (Egan, 1986). It is often useful to point out to clients how much of this they do spontaneously when listening to the therapist. These nonverbal behaviors can be presented both as helping convey the message that they are listening and as actually helping them "tune in" to their partner more effectively (cf. Egan, 1986). When aspects of nonverbal behaviors are very negative, they may be the primary focus of feedback from the therapist. Most commonly, however, we have found it sufficient to mention them in addition to verbal behaviors, which more typically constitute the primary focus of the therapist's attention.

In addition to these very concrete nonverbal listening behaviors, we also encourage spouses to use silence at times to convey attention. In particular, it can be helpful for nondepressed spouses to know that they do not always need to "have an answer" for everything their depressed spouse tells them. Rather, at times they may convey more interest and receptiveness by remaining relaxed and maintaining an attentive focus on the other while saying nothing.

## ATTITUDINAL ISSUES

It is sometimes possible to provide feedback to couples that has to do with adopting an attitude of listening. The goals of good listening can be presented as hearing and showing one has heard, understanding and showing one has understood, empathizing and showing that one can empathize, and acknowledging or showing appreciation to the spouse. These goals imply an active rather than passive stance for the listener and a focus on finding areas of overlap and agreement, rather than an attempt to object to what is being said or to defend oneself. When couples can accept these goals as valid and appropriate, it facilitates their acceptance of the more specific skills discussed below.

## SUMMARIZING

Summarizing simply refers to the act of repeating, in one's own words, the message one believes the partner is trying to convey. The summary statement should always be followed by an inquiry as to whether it was accurate. The following is an example of a typical summary statement from the partner.

BILL: I've been feeling very down lately. The job is really getting to me because it's so menial and so far below my level. And we've been getting along very poorly. The fight at your parents' house on Christmas Eve really depressed me.

SHARON: So it sounds like both the job and our relationship problems have been contributing to your feeling really depressed. Is that right?

At this point, Bill could further emphasize that it was the fight on Christmas Eve that was making him feel bad, or he could say that Sharon had done an accurate job of summarizing his comments. The conversation could then continue, with Bill continuing to be the speaker and Sharon continuing to summarize until he was done with his message. Then Sharon could be the speaker and Bill would summarize her statements.

The most common problem clients have with the summarizing is that they find it to be unnatural. They will resist acting as listeners and attempt to respond with their own comments rather than with a summary of the speaker's message. We emphasize that it is only unnatural because it is not a habit they have right now and because they have not yet made it their own. We predict that over time it will come to feel "right" as well as helping them make the speaker feel heard and understood. At first, we ask couples to summarize almost every message their partner says. As their communication improves, however, summary statements are likely to be necessary less often during a conversation.

## REFLECTING

The skill of reflection is similar to summarizing, but with an additional, more difficult aspect. Whereas summarizing requires only that the listener repeat the significant aspects of the speaker's message, reflection requires that they perceive or infer the speaker's emotional tone as well and perhaps go a little beyond what was said. Because it requires inference, a reflective statement requires interpersonal perceptiveness and sensitivity. Accordingly, there will be individual differences in the ability to learn this skill quickly and efficiently. When working on summarizing, we typically continue until both spouses are proficient. However, for reflecting skills we have found that it is usually sufficient to enhance clients' abilities to reflect accurately until they begin to plateau. Regardless of absolute level of skill attained, when spouses seem unable to perceive affect any more accurately despite several different examples and corrections, this appears to be a reasonable signal that it is time to move on in therapy. We have found it easier to work within a spouse's limitations than to repeat examples and practice *ad infinitum* with little hope of additional gain. A statement and reflective response are given below:

BRIAN: It's just everything at once. It's you, and your coldness to me, it's the possibility of being laid off, it's Katie's problems in school.
SALLY: It sounds like all the problems at once are making you feel overwhelmed, and a little scared. Is that right?

Reflective statements have the ability to help the speaker feel deeply understood and cared for if they are accurate and stated tentatively and with caring. If they are inaccurate or stated as though they were fact, they can backfire. Look at the different effect of the "reflective" statement below, as compared with the one given above.

BRIAN: It's just everything at once. It's you, and your coldness to me, it's the possibility of being laid off, it's Katie's problems in school.
SALLY: You're just feeling scared.

Although it may be true that Brian is scared, the abrupt manner in which Sally stated it made her sound as though she were dismissing his problems rather than empathizing with them. In this example the therapist would comment on the use of the word *just*, suggest elaboration of the feeling expressed by the spouse, and suggest allowing the spouse to comment on whether the reflection was accurate or not.


## VALIDATING

Validation, like reflection, is a difficult listener skill. Some spouses may never learn to validate their spouse when they disagree with him/her. Validation is worth the attempt to teach it, however, because, particularly for depressed couples, being validated by one's spouse is a very positive and relationship-enhancing experience and directly increases the perceived acceptance of emotional expression.

Validation refers to the act of stating that, given the speaker's assumptions, their actions or feelings are legitimate or valid or understandable. It does not require agreement with the stated actions or feelings. Validation statements indicate that the speaker is a worthwhile person acting in an understandable manner (Gottman et al., 1976). A validation sequence is given below:

JANE: When you told me you weren't coming home for supper, I thought it was because you would rather spend time with John and Lou than with me. That's why I was feeling so depressed when you came home.

STEVEN: Well, I can understand why you felt low if you thought I was choosing them and rejecting you. [Note that Steven did not agree with Jane's conclusion that he was rejecting her. He simply validated her feelings, given her assumptions. Contrast this with the more typical disagreement statement likely to ensue following a depressive utterance like Jane's, such as, "That's ridiculous. I simply had to work late."]

Other key phrases besides "I can understand that" in validation statements are, "It makes sense to me," "I see how you felt that way," "You had a right to do that," or "I would have done the same thing in your position." It is not always necessary for these phrases to be spoken, of course, in order for a person to feel validated. Sometimes just listening intently, nodding one's head, and keeping eye contact and body posture warm and open will be sufficient to indicate validation to the listener. Certainly the nonverbal communication must be kept neutral or positive for "validating" phrases to have the desired impact.

The distinction between validation and agreement cannot be overstated, because nearly every client has some difficulty with this point. One can validate another person more easily when one agrees with the other, but validation can be done without agreement (and is much more powerful when it is done during disagreements). In order to successfully validate when one disagrees with the speaker, information regarding the assumptions that led the speaker to act or feel as he/she did must be gathered. Thus the listener who does not understand the speaker's actions or feelings must ask questions to gather sufficient information to validate the speaker.

JANE: I was so depressed when you finally came home last night.

STEVEN: Was there a specific reason? I thought the past few days had gone really well for us.

JANE: When you told me you weren't going to be home for supper, I guess I assumed you preferred the company of John and Lou to me.

STEVEN: Well, I can see how you felt down if you believed that I was rejecting your company in order to be with John and Lou.

## QUESTION ASKING

As can be seen from the above section on validation, communication can often be derailed simply because of a lack of information. It is impossible to reflect or validate another person's statements if one does not have enough information to understand why that person is feeling or acting as he/she is. The most common practice we encounter with question asking is that clients attempt to turn questions into statements. They ask rhetorical questions that are not expected to elicit new information but instead are intended to make a point (e.g., "How in hell was I supposed to get to work if you had the car?"). The nonverbal aspect of communication is very important in question asking. The questioner needs to display genuine interest in and openness to the speaker's response in order for the speaker to feel secure enough to provide the needed information. In the sequence below, we show a good questioner who remains neutral and seeks information when he could easily argue with the points being expressed by his wife (who is not showing particularly good speaker skills). He is attempting to elicit from her the information he needs in order to understand her and therefore to reflect her feelings or to validate her.

SUSAN: I can't believe that you didn't even call me when you were delayed last night. I just felt so lousy waiting for you, waiting and waiting. You are incredibly inconsiderate.

SAM: So it was very upsetting for you waiting for me to come home last night. Why did last night upset you in particular? I've been late a lot in the past few weeks and it didn't seem to bother you.

SUSAN: Last night really got to me because of the argument we had yesterday morning, of course. I felt lousy all day and was really looking forward to seeing you and cooking a nice dinner together. It just felt like you didn't want to be with me or something.

SAM: So did you feel that because I was late I was still mad at you?

SUSAN: Yes, I thought you were punishing me, even though I know you were delayed in traffic and probably couldn't call.

SAM: Look, I can understand how you could feel upset about me being late if you thought I was trying to punish you. Do you still feel that way?

At this point, Sam and Susan can talk about how Sam felt, why he was late, what he did or did not mean by being late. It is very important that the discussion of competing points of view be delayed until the spouse who is upset has had a chance to speak and the partner has, with the aid of appropriate question asking, been able to understand and validate the upset spouse. Only then will the introduction of new information (in this case, what Sam meant by being late) have a positive impact on the communication.

## Speaker Skills to Enhance Empathic Listening

We usually begin by teaching listener skills, despite the fact that they are usually equally poor in speaker and listener skills, because we have found that empathic listening is the area that, if changed, has the greatest impact on the depressive cycle. However, it requires almost superhuman powers to maintain one's empathic listening skills in the face of very poor speaker skills. If the speaker continues to engage in name-calling, derogation, and accusation, continues to be rambling, vague, and agitated, it is highly unlikely that good listening skills will show maintenance over the long run.

    The purpose of teaching speaker skills is to help the clients learn to send clear, specific "I-statements"; send clear, specific requests for change; optimize the content of messages; "edit" out unnecessary negative messages; and keep themselves more calm and relaxed during couple interactions. For depressed clients, sending clear and specific messages is a particularly difficult but important task. Part of the depressed person's difficulties have to do with his/her view of the world in terms of overly negative and absolute categories. It follows that the depressed person also sees the marital difficulties as consisting of nebulous, insurmountable problems. The therapist's job is to teach the client how to label a problem as specifically, clearly, and neutrally as possible. Making this job easier is the fact that couples will have previous experience with being clear and specific from their earlier work on increasing the exchange of positive behavior during the first phase of therapy.

### SENDING CLEAR, SPECIFIC "I-STATEMENTS"

One of the hallmarks of distressed couples in general is that they tend not to take responsibility for their opinions and feelings. Instead, such spouses talk about problems as though their perceptions of their partners' motives and intentions were fact or truth (Noller & Venardos, 1980). Presenting problems in this manner needlessly increases opportunities for misunderstanding and disagreement. For example, two ways of talking about the issue of not putting dirty dishes in the sink would be: (1) "It's so inconsiderate of you to not do that; you're a disgusting slob!" or (2) "When you don't put the dishes in the sink I really feel angry." Both statements are negative in that they express a problem the speaker has with the listener, but in the first, the speaker is focused on "you," the listener, while in the second the speaker is describing how he/she feels, using "I." Talking about one's opinions or feelings in a manner that takes responsibility for them usually requires the use of "I" or "me." Since a statement of how one feels is a statement of fact, not conjecture, couples can learn to use this as a constructive starting point. Misperceptions can be clarified and the "angry" spouse remains more aware of the tentative nature of his/her inferences about the partner. We therefore summarize self-disclosing, responsible statements about problems under the label "I-statements." It is also a cue to the speaker that he/she is getting off track when talking too much about "you."

The use of "I-statements" has several advantages for the communication process. First, it leads to greater self-disclosure by revealing the speaker's preferences, opinions, and feelings in a direct way. This lays the groundwork for increasing felt intimacy in the relationship. Second, it derails the overlearned, negative spousal harangue that is focused on "you." This makes available more functional responses, even in highly emotionally charged situations. Third and perhaps most importantly, it sets the stage for making direct requests of the spouse for assistance in coping with negative situations; that is, it allows the couple to set the stage for joint problem solving.

Clients will often misunderstand and so initially misuse the "I-statement" by putting "I think" or "I feel" on the beginning of a criticism focused on their partner (e.g., "I feel that you have been inconsiderate of me our whole married life; you've never given me the understanding I needed . . . etc."). This, of course, must be noted by the therapist, and feedback should be given as early as possible. It is such a common mistake that we usually predict it when describing what "I-statements" are.

The "formula" we present to clients when talking about problems in terms of "I-statements" is, "When you do $x$ in situation y, I feel $z$" (Lange & Jakubowski, 1976). This formula, while not universally applicable, functions very well as a method of clearly stating one's feelings in response to a partner's actions. It is something for clients to "hang their hat on" and use when they are tempted to simply complain in the old accusatory manner.

"I-statements" are to be used not only for problem descriptions, of course. We especially encourage the use of "I-statements" for communicating positive messages. In this way, the training remains "expressiveness" training rather than becoming overfocused on assertion only. Men especially tend to have difficulty articulating positive feelings in a way that makes their wives feel intimate with them. "I-statements" are very powerful as positive communications. "I love you," "I felt so happy when you said that," "I can't wait for you to get home"—all can be positive disclosures very conducive to the enhancement of positive feelings and the development of greater intimacy.

## SENDING CLEAR, SPECIFIC REQUESTS FOR CHANGE

In order for a request to a partner to change his/her behavior to be effective, it is necessary that the speaker be able to state the problem in clear and specific terms. A request to "be more understanding" may not be acted on, not because the partner is unwilling to change but because he/she may really not know what the speaker means by "more understanding." "When I get home late because I'm stuck in traffic, I would really like it if you could be warm and welcoming to me," is a more specific request that is more likely to get some results.

We train clients in how to make their requests clear and specific by asking them to think about what change in their partner's behavior would make the most difference to them on a particular issue. Frequently, clients need help in thinking about problems in terms of change. Many couples we see are stuck in a complaining cycle. They complain to each other endlessly, usually over the same things, but never make a specific request for change. Global, chronic complaints tend to make the listener "turn off," whereas specific requests for change are much more manageable and less likely to be immediately rejected by the listener. Much of our time with clients on this issue is spent asking the question, "And what would you like from him (her)?" We hope the clients will eventually internalize this question. To help them internalize it, we regularly interject such comments as, "No one can have more access to what you want than you do; therefore, if you have difficulty saying exactly what you want, imagine how much harder it must be for your spouse to figure it out." Thus it becomes each individual's responsibility to clarify for him/herself and then for the spouse exactly what is needed from the other.

Learning how to request change from a partner is a therapeutic task that goes to the heart of the depression/marital discord interaction. Depressed persons do not tend to see their problems as changeable and therefore are unlikely to think in terms of what changes they would like. Moreover, the type of marital situation conducive to depression is one in which requests for change may have been ignored in the past. Thus, if the therapist can succeed in getting depressed clients to make specific, calm requests for change from their partners (to which the partners respond), a major therapeutic goal has been achieved.

## OPTIMIZING MESSAGE CONTENT

Two of the biggest problems we have seen with the message content of distressed, depressed couples are that they ramble on too long and are not clear enough in what they say. These two problems are related. If clients can be taught to be concise, their clarity also increases greatly. This problem is at the heart of many complaints that the spouse never listens. Frequently when one partner complains of not being listened to, it is the case that he/she is indeed difficult to listen to. The problem can be further exacerbated by the natural tendency to explain more and go on longer when it appears that the partner does not understand.

Being concise is a remarkably difficult skill to teach to some people. Some individuals we worked with never succeeded at shortening their own utterances but did at least learn to accept feedback from the spouse, such as "I think I know what you are saying; please let me speak now." The better the partner is at summarizing, reflecting, and validating, the easier time the garrulous partner has at becoming succinct, because he/she will feel heard.

## EDITING UNNECESSARY NEGATIVE MESSAGES

The skill of knowing what *not* to say is at least as important as the other speaker skills. Accompanying the theme of keeping messages concise and specific is the idea that there are many utterances that will not help the communication process. Gottman et al. (1976) call the skill of not saying unnecessary negative things "editing." They also have an apt descriptive term for the opposite, filling a discussion with extraneous negatives. They call this "kitchen sinking," that is, throwing in everything but the kitchen sink. The result of kitchen sinking is rarely a positive resolution of an issue. Much more frequently, bringing up more than one negative topic is a recipe for an unproductive argument. We attempt to train our couples to edit out unnecessary negatives by getting them to focus on what they want from the discussion.

## REMAINING CALM AND RELAXED
## DURING COUPLE DISCUSSIONS

For couples who have a pattern of loud, angry, escalating arguments, a major focus of communication training should be on how to maintain a more neutral emotional tone, even when discussing problem topics. These couples have developed an escalation pattern in which the anger or irritation of one partner serves as a trigger for further anger on the part of the other partner, and so on. Couples with this problem need specific training in maintaining emotional control. If they are not able to discuss even minor problems without escalating anger, they may require more formal anger-control training (e.g., Novaco, 1979).

We have found that much of the overemotionality in depressed, discordant couples is associated with long histories of poor communication in which the partners experienced extreme frustration when attempting to influence each other. If the therapist can aid such a couple with effective communication strategies—especially calm, attentive listening— then the overemotionality may subside. In any case, the therapist should make it clear that emotional neutrality in problem discussions is very helpful in bringing about positive resolution of difficulties.

## Increasing the Frequency and Breadth of Intimate Exchanges

In the context of improved listening and speaking skills, an increased ability to speak directly to the spouse, and a calmer, more cohesive atmosphere, there is an opportunity to begin to facilitate the occurrence of greater intimacy in the dyad. Several factors are of primary importance in facilitating intimacy. First, the level of attraction and liking between the partners should have begun to increase. Liking tends to facilitate increased self-disclosure, and self-disclosure can, in turn, help partners feel closer and more intimate (Taylor, 1979). Second, it should be clear that both spouses have the necessary skills to listen appropriately to self-disclosures from their partner. There is little point in suggesting that couples self-disclose when they lack the prerequisite listening skills to make this a positive experience. Third, it may be necessary to create settings that are conducive to increased breadth and depth of self-disclosure. In particular, it may be necessary to reconstruct or enhance family and couple activities that provide relaxed, low-demand opportunities to share information about the day and ongoing events and feelings. Fourth, it is likely to be important to specifically encourage *positive* self-disclosure. It is positive self-disclosure that is most likely to lead to reciprocity from the spouse and become self-sustaining.

## The Role of Increased Liking

As spouses find themselves doing more together and enjoying each other more, it is usual for them to have somewhat more positive feelings toward each other. They may also find that they share common interests and values. Both these factors should increase spouses' willingness to self-disclose to each other. Typically, this increased self-disclosure will first take the form of increased discussion of everyday matters and matters of shared interest, such as children, neighborhood, extended family, household, friends, daily events, plans for upcoming events, or reminiscence about previous experiences. If these disclosures are received well, self-disclosure will begin to deepen into the sharing of positive feelings toward the spouse, statements about closeness and commitment, a willingness to self-disclose thoughts and reactions to events, and reciprocated self-disclosures. As the overall amount of self-disclosure increases, it is likely that spouses will notice that they are beginning to experience some excitement or strong feelings during episodes in which high levels of self-disclosure occur (cf. Beach & Tesser, 1987). To the extent that these feelings are frightening to either the depressed or nondepressed spouse, they sometimes need to be discussed directly as a possible obstacle to further progress. However, increased cohesion and liking often lead to increased breadth of self-disclosure with little additional therapeutic intervention required.

## The Role of Listening Skills

The skills of empathic listening are all likely to come into play in the context of self-disclosure. It is through the use of these skills that the spouse can reward and encourage self-disclosure and so help maintain its occurrence. In addition, when spouses are adept at reflection, validation, and question asking, they can powerfully convey the message of acceptance and encouragement of self-disclosure. It is typically best, however, when both spouses feel free to take the role of discloser as well as that of listener. Unreciprocated self-disclosure is characteristic of nonegalitarian relationships and may tend to exacerbate feelings of distance in the relationship rather than increase feelings of closeness.

## Creating or Reconstructing Settings for Self-Disclosure

The best setting for self-disclosure is likely to be one in which the individual feels safe and comfortable. It is possible that this includes physical as well as psychological comfort (Chaikin, Derlega, & Miller, 1976). Thus it is important that the couple be encouraged to share relaxed time in a comfortable setting. It will often be the case that this has already occurred as a byproduct of earlier successes in increasing cohesion. However, sometimes couples will have increased cohesion by engaging in activities that are active and enjoyable, but do not promote conversation and verbal interaction. Indeed, some couples will be entirely lacking in the "usual" settings for self-disclosure, such as shared mealtimes, discussions in bed before going to sleep, shared evening events at home not involving the television, coffee or tea times, or other regular daily times for low-key conversation and interaction. When such settings are lacking, but other conditions appear promising, it makes sense for the therapist to begin to encourage the development of new daily routines for the couple that produce such settings.

## Encouraging Positive Self-Disclosure

While it is very important that couples be able to tolerate negative self-disclosure and deal with it constructively, negative self-disclosures cannot be expected to deepen feelings of intimacy (Chelune, Sultan, Vosk, Ogden, & Waring, 1984; Tolstedt & Stokes, 1984). Even after working to establish the appropriate relationship context and settings for self-disclosure, the therapist must therefore be alert to the possibility that self-disclosures will be predominantly negative, thus tending to punish the developing pattern of self-disclosure rather than rewarding and maintaining it. It is sometimes necessary in this context to work directly with spouses on expressing positive feelings and observations to each other. It should be acknowledged at the outset that this will be somewhat difficult for the depressed spouse, since he/she will be prone to recall negative events more readily. However, it is usually possible to build on earlier work aimed at increasing compliments and praise given to the spouse as well as work aimed at using "I-statements" for the expression of positive feelings to encourage continued self-disclosure of positive feelings in a genuine manner. An added benefit of greater self-disclosure of positive feelings and observations is that it promotes positive tracking and increased mutual reinforcement of positive behavior in the relationship.

## Enhancing Perceived and Actual Coping Assistance: A Focus on Problem-Solving Training

One of the greatest factors influencing the actual coping support forthcoming from the spouse as well as the perceived availability of coping support from the spouse is the extent to which spouses can engage in resolving problems jointly and constructively. Problem-solving training can help to increase the ability of the partners to provide this kind of concrete aid to each other.

Before we train couples in problem solving, we attempt to have them discriminate between the two major reasons for communication in marriage. One is to solve a problem. The other is simply to express oneself to an intimate other (cf. Weiss, 1978). The listener and sender skills outlined above are necessary for both types of communication. However, not all discussions that include some negative content need be problem-solving sessions. There is an important role for simple communication of feelings in developing a more intimate relationship. This distinction is of particular concern with our depressed, discordant couples. A common dysfunction for discordant, depressed couples begins with one partner (usually the depressed one) trying to express some negative feelings, hoping for some understanding and validation from the other. The partner then responds with an unwanted problem-solving approach: giving advice or suggestions about what the speaker can do to avoid these negative feelings in the future. The interaction ends with the speaker feeling misunderstood and the listener feeling frustrated in his/her attempt to help the speaker. Both partners are trying hard to communicate, but they are missing the boat because they focused on different functions of communication.

To avoid these problems, we teach couples to identify the type of communication they want. If the speaker wants to solve a problem, he/she is taught to articulate that to the other partner (e.g., "I'd like your help in figuring out what to do about the situation in the office"). Similarly, if the speaker simply wants to share some feelings, that should also be articulated up front (e.g., "I've been feeling really down; can I just get a sympathetic ear?"). After learning more basic empathic listening and speaker skills, the couple is typically in a good position to make this discrimination.

When is problem solving necessary? Problem solving is necessary when a couple encounters a situation in which clear expressions of each person's wishes do not suffice to resolve a conflict. We have found that a good foundation in the speaker and listener skills outlined above, coupled with the ability to neutralize the emotional tone of discussions, is sufficient to reduce the number of conflicts within the dyad. Because many conflicts are triggered by trivial issues, it is the process of communication, rather than its content, that leads to the conflict. However, there remain those disagreements that are unsolvable without using the techniques of problem solving.

## Attitudinal Issues in Problem Solving

Couple-oriented problem solving is predicated on several beliefs. First, problems constitute a normal part of married life. Thus it is not the discovery or perception of a relationship problem that is troublesome, but rather the response to it. A difficulty recognized and dealt with in a joint, constructive manner need present no problems for a relationship. Second, marital problems have solutions (or at least partial solutions), and such solutions are worth searching for. Third, when one identifies a problem in the relationship it is appropriate to avoid acting on impulse and instead to bring the issue to a joint problem-solving discussion. Fourth, any problem resolution in which one partner "loses" is not actually a "win" for the other partner, since in a marriage the happiness of each depends on the happiness of the other. In other words, in attempting problem resolutions, a "win–win" solution is always preferable.

## Course of Training in Problem Solving

As in all our communication skills training, we attempt to maximize success experiences by starting with easier tasks and progressing to more difficult ones. We first give clients a short handout describing problem solving and provide them an overview of what we will cover. Then we employ an imaginary problem in practicing the skills (i.e., we choose a problem that is a significant marital issue for some people but that does not happen to trouble this couple). This use of an imaginary rather than a real problem early in problem-solving training serves several functions. First, it enables the couple to focus on the techniques of problem solving rather than being swept up in the content of the problem being discussed. Second, using a problem that they themselves do not have can make a couple feel good about their strengths, since they implicitly compare themselves to couples who have the problem. Third, because an imaginary problem does not carry with it learned emotional responses, the couple has a better chance of coming up with some solutions than they would if they were to use a real problem.

After a couple has succeeded in "solving" an imaginary problem, the therapist can help them choose a relatively nonemotional real problem to attempt to solve. Ideal problems at this stage are "practical" in nature—issues such as what car to buy, where to go on vacation, or what color to paint their living room can be good choices *if* they have not been points of contention in the past. Only after couples have succeeded at both imaginary and practical problems are they ready to attempt using problem solving on emotion-laden topics.

## Outline of Problem Solving

We teach our clients a slightly modified version of the D'Zurilla and Goldfried (1971) model of problem solving. Considerable useful detail on problem solving as a therapeutic modality can also be found in D'Zurilla (1988) and Nezu and colleagues (1989). There are six stages involved.

### PROBLEM DEFINITION

This stage is particularly important for depressed, discordant couples. Perceiving the world as consisting of overwhelming difficulties, they therefore talk about problems in global terms. "We can't communicate" is far too global to be considered a well-defined problem. The therapist is always working to help couples make their complaints concrete and specific. In problem solving, the entire procedure is predicated on good problem definition. A well-defined problem should be concrete and specific and also include the problem from both partners' point of view. For example, "When I'm feeling down, like I was over the weekend, I want to be able to share my feelings with you, but you seem to feel very angry and upset when I talk about being depressed. So the problem is how can we communicate when I'm feeling down so that I feel understood and you are not made unhappy. Do you agree?" Clients are coached in being as specific as possible and stating the problem in a way that includes *both* partners' needs or desires.

### BRAINSTORMING

The second stage is one that most people normally do not include in their problem-solving routine. Brainstorming simply means generating many possible solutions, with no restrictions on how impractical or silly they may be. The idea is to loosen up the thinking process by separating the problem-generation phase from the evaluation phase. The therapist must urge clients to refrain from evaluation (e.g., "No, you know we can't possibly do that") when brainstorming is occurring. This can also be a time to lighten up the problem discussion by suggesting impractical solutions, which may nonetheless contain a grain of truth that could be transformed into a real solution. For example, when brainstorming on the issue of how to spend more time together, a husband suggested "sending the children away to boarding school." Although the couple laughed at this because it was not at all within their financial grasp, it led the wife to suggest asking her parents to take the kids for a week during the summer, a practical suggestion that they did in fact implement.

## SOLUTION EVALUATION

In order for solution evaluation to go well, it is important for the couple to have internalized the "win–win" philosophy articulated above. The evaluation must include the effects of the solution on both parties. We have couples give a percentage score to each solution in terms of how much it satisfies the desires of each partner, with 100% being perfectly satisfactory to both, 50% being either perfectly satisfactory to one and not at all satisfactory to the other or somewhat satisfactory to both, and so on. In this way, couples are aided in learning to evaluate solutions with an eye to mutual satisfaction. Couples often need help in identifying and rating the various costs and benefits of each solution.

## SOLUTION SELECTION

Once couples have discussed their desires and rated solutions, they need to select a solution to try out. If their evaluation has been done well, with an emphasis on mutual satisfaction and maximizing benefits over costs, then the selection should be relatively straightforward. It is important, however, to get couples to make a firm agreement about what they are going to do before they terminate the problem-solving discussion. The selection of a solution, therefore, should include discussion of how it is to be done. For example, if a couple has decided that the best way to solve their problem of not doing enough enjoyable things on the weekend is to make plans for the weekend by the previous Wednesday, then before they terminate the discussion they must decide who is to make plans this week and how they will select who makes plans in any given week.

## SOLUTION ENACTMENT

Finally, the couples must act on the agreement for change. This stage may be particularly problematic for depressed couples, since they are typically lethargic and feel hopeless about the possibility of change

through action. Couples must be coached through this stage and encouraged in the belief that trying out a solution, any solution, is preferable to
inaction.

## OUTCOME EVALUATION

This stage requires the therapist's help in teaching clients not to throw the
baby out with the bath water; that is, partial failures must be examined
for what went right as well as what went wrong and how it can be
improved. Depressive clients tend to evaluate situations in black-and-
white terms, a tendency that can be disruptive of problem solving. It is
not uncommon for clients to say, after one failure in problem solving,
"Problem solving doesn't work for us." Of course, they must learn to
produce more fine-grained evaluations and, most important, to try, try
again.

# Enhancing the Perception
# of Spousal Dependability

Many of the discordant, depressed couples we have worked with directly
or indirectly raised concerns about the stability of their marriage or at
least the stability of their partner's intent to continue investing energy in
improving the relationship. Often these concerns are expressed in the
context of a perceived lack of commitment to the marriage by one or
both of the spouses. These concerns can engender serious problems
regarding the perception of spousal dependability, a key area if gains
made in marital therapy are going to translate into long-term gains in
symptom-free functioning. In addition, Beach and Tesser (1987) have
hypothesized that where commitment to the marriage truly is low one can
expect an erosion over time in cohesion, as spouses decrease the amount
of attention they give to relationship issues, as well as an erosion over
time in intimacy, as spouses become increasingly reluctant to trust and
take chances with their partner. Thus commitment and the perception of
spousal commitment must be of concern to the marital therapist working
with a discordant, depressed population. In addition, it is not uncommon
for spouses to point to prior events in the relationship that seem to
suggest that the partner is not trustworthy or is unlikely to follow
through on verbal commitments. In these situations, the therapist must
be ready to modify dysfunctional attributions for prior spousal behavior
or help the couple allay these concerns in some other way to prevent them

from unnecessarily compromising the depressed spouse's ability to benefit from increased marital satisfaction.

## Increasing the Less Committed Spouse's Commitment

One of the most important variables related to increasing commitment to the relationship—increasing the rewards derived from the relationship—will have already been attended to by the midphase of therapy (Thibaut & Kelley, 1959). From the perspective of social exchange theory, interventions discussed previously in the context of enhancing cohesion and self-esteem support or increasing positive events in the relationship can be seen as influencing level of commitment as well. In addition, as positive events within the marriage come to be more salient for each spouse, it is likely that perceptions of personal commitment will increase. Our experience is that many couples do experience marked increases in felt commitment as a result of other interventions in therapy without direct intervention regarding commitment per se.

Sometimes, however, couples will appear to be making changes in the areas of increasing cohesion, enhancing communication skills, and increasing the frequency of positive events within the relationship without a corresponding increase in the apparent long-term commitment of the initially less committed spouse. One common problem in these cases is that the more committed spouse (often the depressed partner) is overfocused on the marital relationship as the source of all gratification. As Stuart (1980) has pointed out, this exclusive focus on the marriage by one partner can actually contribute to the *lower* commitment of the other. In particular, it can lead the less committed spouse to devalue the need for acting committed, since it seems so clear the partner will not leave in any case. Moreover, when the partner is overfocused on obtaining relationship rewards, the less committed spouse may also find him/ herself in the position of continually limiting the amount of time spent together. Through a process of self-perception (Bem, 1972), this can lead to the conclusion that "I must not be very committed to the relationship."

We have found that increased commitment is sometimes forthcoming in such cases when the wife is supported in the decision to seek outside employment or to increase individual outside pleasant activities. In many cases this appears to make the committed partner more interesting and to stimulate increased attention from the previously less committed partner. As suggested by Stuart (1980), it may also create a climate of increased uncertainty for the previously less committed spouse that has the effect of increasing arousal and the strength of positive emotions.

The therapist may have the opportunity to directly influence other beliefs relevant to commitment during the course of therapy. In particular, the therapist often has opportunities to make more salient the costs of leaving an ongoing relationship or the rewards to be lost by leaving the relationship. According to social exchange theory, as these factors become more salient to the individual there should be a corresponding increase in felt commitment.

## Enhancing the Perception of the Spouse as Committed

It is often difficult for spouses to accurately gauge their partner's level of commitment. Since commitment is primarily defined in terms of a nonevent (i.e., not leaving the relationship) or future events (e.g., will continue to invest in the relationship 2 years from now), this should not be surprising. It is well known that individuals have great difficulty in assimilating information conveyed via nonevents (Nisbett & Ross, 1980). Thus one spouse may continue to view the other as uncommitted even though the other appears to have made a strong investment in the relationship and appears to be willing to continue investing. In these cases, it may be appropriate for the therapist to begin to encourage the spontaneous expression of feelings of commitment as a way of making commitment more observable. Changes in routine or in the relationship may also be labeled as indications of commitment. The goal in these cases is to provide enough evidence of observable behavior capable of being interpreted as "committed behavior" that it can successfully challenge the belief that the spouse remains uncommitted. When both spouses believe that their partner is committed, this increases trust and further facilitates positive change in the dyad.

## Restructuring Dysfunctional Attributions for Prior Spousal Behavior

On occasion, it is particularly difficult to increase the perception of the spouse as committed because prior behavior has been inconsistent or ambiguous. The most typical example will involve spouses who have attempted to change before and have resolved their difficulties, only to find them returning again a short while later. It is not uncommon in these cases for one spouse to blame the other for the return of the problem and to see this as evidence that the partner "cannot keep a promise," or "is too lazy to really change," or "is only pretending to change." In these cases it may be necessary to address directly the spouse's negative attributions for the previous behavior.

One model that may be of help in addressing problems of this type is the attribution-efficacy model (Fincham & Bradbury, 1987b; Fincham et al., 1990). This model suggests that it may be possible to disrupt entrenched attributions of blame by addressing judgments of causal stability, globality, and whether the cause of the event was really something about the partner. In particular, it is possible to formulate plausible causes of the problem that are specific to the past and no longer pertain, or would be expected to affect only a particular set of problems that this couple has already resolved, or involve clear external stressors or obstacles that are either no longer present or are more easily coped with at present. In this way, the fact that there have been problems in the past need not result in the conclusion that it was all the partner's fault, or that it will happen again, or that all attempts at change are equally doomed to failure. The attribution-efficacy model also suggests that entrenched blame may be disrupted by helping spouses dispute the supposed voluntariness of the behavior in question, the presumed motivation of the behavior, or the intent of the behavior. In particular, it is important to examine previous problems to determine whether they can be seen as having been involuntary, motivated by prosocial or benign motives, or derived from the intent to produce a positive outcome. If so, a situation previously seen as a cause for blame and evidence of the spouse's lack of dependability can be reinterpreted as being largely irrelevant to the current changes the couple is making, or perhaps even evidence of their long-standing mutual involvement, the stability of their relationship regardless of what else was happening in the relationship, and their mutual commitment. While this is not suggested for every case, it can be a particularly useful strategy for couples who are otherwise good responders to therapy but cannot quite believe it will last.

## Decreasing Stressors during the Middle Stage of Therapy

The majority of our work with depressed, discordant couples involves teaching them skills (such as problem-solving and communication skills) that we hope they can carry with them when therapy ends. When recurrent stressful patterns are identified during the middle stage of therapy, these will most typically be used as examples of issues for problem-solving interaction. However, we have found that some issues are relatively straightforward from the therapist's perspective, and in these cases we sometimes will assign outright attempts to change behavior. The decision to take this approach will typically result from the therapist's perception that there are many other issues that represent good opportunities for problem solving and that this particular problem area might go unaddressed in therapy if it were to be dealt with in a problem-solving mode. In addition, it will typically be the case that leaving the stressor unaddressed appears to pose a problem for the process of change in the couple.

An example of direct therapist intervention to reduce a stressor can be found in the case of a couple we saw who were having inordinate difficulty driving together on trips. Debbie resented having to be the navigator; she wanted her husband, Scott, to pay attention and drive without her assistance and constant reminders of directions. Scott agreed he would not ask for her help; but when he did not ask, he would frequently make mistakes and take them slightly out of their way. Therefore Debbie continued her angry "helping" because she felt trapped by Scott's "ineptitude" with directions. The therapist saw a mutually determined pattern: Debbie expected Scott to show perfect competence immediately in tasks that had been her exclusive domain for years, and Scott's fear of Debbie's anger if he were not perfect made him reluctant to try new tasks. They seemed stuck in this pattern, and both believed the problem was unsolvable. The therapist gave them the assignment of having Scott exclusively in charge of directions. Debbie was to say nothing at all regarding directions, even if Scott tried to enlist her help. She was also to say nothing if Scott made a mistake and took them out of their way. It was emphasized that they both had their tasks to work on and that both were difficult. Scott had to take responsibility for directions, which required him to study the map beforehand and to keep alert on the road. Debbie had to keep calm and relaxed and let Scott do what she claimed she wanted him to do: take control.

The above assignment worked well for Debbie and Scott. The reason the therapist assigned this to them rather than having them problem solve on the issue was that they had shown that they each saw the problem as insoluble. Thus it would have been very difficult to gain their compliance with a problem-solving format. Even had they agreed to a problem-solving format, it seemed unlikely that they would come up with a workable solution. Although they did not practice problem solving in the context of this problem, they did learn that even problems they initially saw as unsolvable could have solutions. Thus, when they express doubts about being able to solve a particular problem, it was possible to reflect on this example and help them establish a better general orientation to problem solving. While this type of directive problem solving by the therapist can clearly be overdone to the detriment of therapy, we believe that it also has its place in the therapy process.

## Working on Special Problem Areas

Couples present with a variety of concerns in addition to their concerns about their marriage and about the depression being experienced by one or both spouses. Concerns may be raised about long-standing sexual difficulties, such as anorgasmia or erectile problems. Concerns may be expressed about previous episodes of extramarital sexual relationships or prior episodes in which one spouse left the home for some period of time. During routine assessment, issues of one or both spouses' use of drugs and/or alcohol may emerge as salient problem areas. Likewise, it is not uncommon for couples to have questions about how best to handle problems their children are experiencing. In each of these cases the therapist will need to determine the relative importance of working on one problem as opposed to another. In every case, the therapist will need to realize that not all problems can be worked on at the same time. Therefore the therapist and the couple need to agree on the order in which problems should be addressed. Most typically, we have found that it is easier to address sexual problems after other problems in the marriage and with depression have begun to improve. Conversely, where physical abuse is an issue, we have often found it necessary to deal with the abuse at the outset of therapy. Likewise, when alcohol or drugs are being used in a very abusive manner, this pattern may need to be among the first issues addressed. Whenever auxiliary issues are to be dealt with in therapy, the therapist must make a clinical decision about the needs of the particular couple and the way in which the auxiliary issues can best be dealt with. It is probably never appropriate to simply assume that these other problems will disappear entirely once the marital problems have been adequately resolved. Rather, it may often be necessary to extend the course of therapy to allow a focus on these issues either before or after working on improving the marital relationship in general.

## Process Issues in Midtherapy

We have found several issues that tend to come up in the middle phase of therapy. We have found it helpful to attend to these issues and to deal with them as soon as they appear.

## Midtherapy Decrease in Motivation

Data from our outcome study provide some documentation that there is a dip in marital satisfaction in the middle phase of therapy, after a rapid increase in satisfaction during the early stage (see Figure 6-2). We have hypothesized that this dip occurs because there is a decrease in morale when the therapeutic focus shifts from increasing positives (as outlined in Chapter 5) to dealing with longer-standing problems. This is a sensitive period in terms of overall therapeutic gains, because couples must overcome this initial reaction to dealing with unpleasant problems in order to show lasting improvement.

This pattern has proven so common that we now predict it to couples. We tell them that it is understandable that they will feel temporarily less motivated and less happy together as we begin to work on problems. We emphasize that most couples overcome these initial feelings and go on to make additional gains in their marital satisfaction. Most importantly, we request that couples be compliant with homework assignments *even though* they may initially feel as though their marital problems are hopeless or overwhelming.

## Unequal Effort between Partners

By the middle phase of therapy, it sometimes becomes quite apparent that one partner is working significantly less hard at making changes in the relationship. Understandably, this can decrease the motivation of the hard-working partner and can itself be a cause of discord and depression. The reasons for this discrepancy must be carefully analyzed by the therapist. Sometimes noncompliance by one spouse is a nonverbal message to the therapist that his/her needs are not being met by the therapy so far. Other times, noncompliance is a message that the relationship is not as important to one spouse as it is to the other. This is frequently the case when one spouse has already made a covert decision to pursue divorce or, less commonly, is engaged in an undisclosed extramarital affair. We have usually found it most helpful and least disruptive to the therapy to confront individuals separately on any issue that is not symmetrical and/or that may involve "secrets." While some writers in the field urge couples therapists never to see the individuals alone for fear of becoming party to secrets that cannot be shared with the other spouse, we have found it impossible to work with noncompliant spouses without individual sessions. To confront only one member of a couple in a conjoint session violates the symmetry rule that is essential to maintaining both partners' view of therapist fairness. If we find out a "secret" in such an individual session, we urge the spouse to share it and offer our help in doing so. We would not continue conjoint therapy with a couple in which one partner has made a firm decision to leave the relationship. However, we would attempt to convince a partner who is ambivalent about the marriage to increase his/her compliance as the only fair way of investigating whether this relationship can succeed. We tell such individuals that divorce can always be chosen after therapy has ended if they are not satisfied with the relationship at that time.

We are very sensitive to the danger of keeping a depressed person in marital therapy with a noncompliant spouse. It is a destructive and depressing experience to be trying to change one's relationship and to have one's partner doing nothing. We feel it is preferable to engage the depressed person in individual therapy from the outset if his/her spouse is likely not to comply in couples therapy. However, if couples therapy has already been started and noncompliance then emerges, then the actions outlined above should be considered.

## Confrontation with a Partner's Limited Capacities

When one partner appears to be doing less than the other partner, this is sometimes a matter of limited capacities rather than limited motivation. During the mid- to late therapy phase, spouses can see how much change their partner is capable of. Sometimes this can be disappointing. As one woman, Anne, said to her therapist, "I know Ralph has changed some things about himself that have bothered me, and I think he has tried, but he is just never going to be the kind of sensitive, expressive person I would like him to be." After seeing real effort and change in their partners and their relationship, some individuals are struck by the partners' relative incapacity to achieve the kind of change they had fantasized about. We have found that a few sessions of individual therapy focused on holding realistic expectations of their partners can be helpful to such individuals.

## Case Example: Mary Jo and Michael

Mary Jo and Michael were a couple in their late 30s who had two small children. They both had strict Catholic upbringing. Mary Jo had been depressed for about 6 months when they started therapy, and both acknowledged that the marriage had never been very good. They were experiencing sexual problems and constant bickering; in addition, they were unable to productively solve major life problems, such as whether Mary Jo should return to school or have a third child. Michael's style was unassertive and passive; he tried to avoid conflict at all costs. Mary Jo, in contrast, was highly emotional and confrontational.

Their first five sessions focused on increasing time together, which was difficult because of their small children and conflicting work schedules. They were also guided in performing caring gestures for one another. The impact of increasing positives was strong for this couple. They entered the second phase of therapy feeling much warmer toward each other. Also, Mary Jo was no longer depressed.

The therapeutic agenda at this time was to help them improve their communication styles so that Michael could be assertive and direct and Mary Jo could be less emotional and aversive during conflict. To this end, the therapy concentrated on helping Michael with speaker skills, helping Mary Jo with emotional self-control, aiding both with empathic listening, and teaching both problem solving.

## Session 6

In session 6, Mary Jo came in complaining vigorously about Michael's unassertive behavior with his parents over the past week. They had asked him to do several favors that Mary Jo regarded as totally outrageous, considering that they had six other children besides Michael. Michael basically agreed that his parents had taken advantage of him. This problem was used as an example in introducing communication skills training. The therapist introduced summarizing and had both parties attempt it during the session, first with the therapist and then with the spouse. Michael was more successful than Mary Jo in the skill. The therapist gave them each feedback about their performance, stressing to Mary Jo that her emotionality was an impediment to the progress of the conversation. They were given the homework assignment of talking further about the same issue at home, maintaining separate speaker and listener roles, and using summarizing. They were instructed to have no more than two such sessions, neither of which was to last longer than 10 minutes. They were asked to tape-record the sessions.

## Session 7

Michael and Mary Jo came into session 7 somewhat downhearted. They felt that the communication session had not gone well, and they were feeling hopeless about their problems once again. They had, fortunately, taped the session. The therapist was therefore able to change the topic from their negative assessment of the week and focus the discussion on analysis of the communication session itself. Before playing the tape, the therapist asked Michael and Mary Jo each to note what they themselves had done wrong and to give a critique of their own behavior. The therapist stopped the tape recorder whenever one of them had said something that seemed detrimental to the communication process. Again, Michael was better than Mary Jo in identifying what he had done wrong. The therapist emphasized the connection between Mary Jo's anger and yelling and the downward spiral of the discussion.

Speaker skills were briefly introduced, including "I-statements," clarity, and the importance of emotional neutrality. Again, the assignment was given to discuss a topic (about a more mundane issue this time—their feelings about a particular babysitter) and to use the skill of summarizing. They were also encouraged to keep up with their positive interactions, which had been abandoned when not specifically assigned.

## Session 8

The couple had not done the homework assignment. Michael said it was because Mary Jo had refused; Mary Jo said she had just been too busy. The therapist suspected she was paying the price (through the couple's noncompliance) for neglecting symmetry in her feedback during the last session, when she had pinpointed Mary Jo's anger and yelling as the prime problem in their disastrous communication attempt. Although this may have been a correct assessment, she had probably alienated Mary Jo somewhat. The therapist therefore attempted to be more symmetrical when giving her feedback to the couple after this, even though she did continue to see Mary Jo as having the greater difficulty with communication.

Since the couple had not done the assignment, the therapist had them tape the assigned communication session while she stepped out of the room (after providing a short refresher on what the assignment was). Then the tape was analyzed with the couple, with each serving as his/her own critic, with guidance from the therapist. The therapist intentionally gave slightly more critical feedback to Michael than she did in the last session.

The second half of the session was spent going over the speaker skill of reflection. It was explained and modeled by the therapist, using an issue brought up by the couple (training their dog). They each attempted it with the therapist role playing the spouse, and both were given feedback. Finally, they attempted it with each other. They were fairly successful, and the therapist praised them for this. They were given the assignment of using both summary and reflection in an at-home discussion and instructed to tape it.

## Session 9

Michael and Mary Jo were both quite pleased with themselves in that they had successfully completed their assignment. They listened to the tape with the therapist, and she pinpointed what they had done right, especially how they had changed for the better in their communication.

The listener skills mentioned briefly in session 7 were brought up again by the therapist, and each partner was asked how good he/she was at that skill. Mary Jo and Michael were both able to be quite accurate in their self-evaluations of clarity and conciseness, taking responsibility, editing out unnecessary negatives, and maintaining a neutral emotional tone. The listener skill of validation was also introduced in this session. Because the couple did not seem to grasp the idea of validation completely, their assignment did not include it; instead they were to begin to talk about their "big issue," which was whether Mary Jo should have another baby. They were warned that this was a very difficult topic and that they were *not* to attempt to solve it; they were only to express themselves clearly and to be good listeners to their partner. The topic of whether or not to have a baby was not thought to be the ideal topic for this stage of their communication training, but they had been wanting to discuss it since the beginning of therapy and had brought it up again during session 9; so the therapist decided it would be counterproductive to postpone it longer.

## Session 10

As expected, the homework session did not go perfectly, but Mary Jo and Michael had made an honest attempt at using their skills on a difficult and emotionally charged issue. The therapist praised them for their positive achievements and emphasized how it would have gone had they not used their skills. She then introduced the steps of problem solving and the rationale of using a systematic method of deciding on a course of action. Since the issue of whether or not to have a baby had already been opened, the couple was very reluctant to use any other topic to "practice" problem solving. The therapist therefore began to go through the stages of problem solving using the baby issue. The assignment was to continue the problem-solving session at home.

## Session 11

They had not gotten far with the problem-solving assignment before it had deteriorated into an emotional argument. The therapist helped them go through the stages of problem solving in session using the baby issue. They were able to do all the stages well except for the solution evaluation. They were both tied into a win–lose mentality. The therapist spent some time discussing with them the effects on the marriage if either person felt truly unhappy with the outcome of the decision, in an attempt to help them see that it was to each one's benefit to make sure the other person was also happy. They were able to accept this. The therapist also helped guide them to a more sensitive evaluation of the issues at stake. Neither Michael nor Mary Jo was as clear about the issue as they were portraying themselves to be. Mary Jo had her own doubts about having another child, and Michael loved children greatly. Michael's main argument against having another baby was that he was worried about financial matters. A tentative solution was proposed: They were going to wait for a year; if Michael's promised raise came through, they would attempt to have another child. If not, they would renegotiate.

# 7

## Ending Therapy: Issues of Maintenance, Disengagement, and Continued Change

Although maintenance of gains is always a concern for therapists, it is even more of a concern when working with a depressed, discordant population. If it is the case that amelioration of marital stressors and improvement in marital sources of support are important for the prevention of future episodes of depression, then a relapse into marital discord is doubly dangerous. It not only represents a relapse in relationship problems but also poses the threat of a relapse in depression for one or both partners. In addition, it increasingly appears that relapse is relatively common at longer lags posttherapy for discordant couples (Jacobson, Schmaling, & Holtzworth-Munroe, 1987). Thus, for this approach to treatment, the issue of relapse must be considered critical and not yet completely resolved.

We have attempted to address the problem of maintenance of gains after marital therapy of depression with several techniques used during the final phase of therapy. These include fading out the directive role of the therapist; narrowing the scope of therapy to the issues that prove to be most important for the particular couple; and reinforcing problem solving as a skill the couple can use to prevent future difficulties or use to continue making positive changes in their relationship. Additionally, we have included a discussion of "booster sessions." Booster sessions are regularly scheduled sessions that take place several weeks or months after the end of therapy. The underlying assumption behind the inclusion of booster sessions is that the use of skills taught in marital therapy for depression is liable to decrease without explicit efforts at renewal. In addition, couples may be vulnerable to external sources of stress that were not envisioned while therapy was ongoing. Thus, booster sessions allow the therapist to continue working with the couple at a much reduced intensity to further facilitate positive change and prevent relapse (Jacobson, 1989).

Attitudes and expectations regarding the end of therapy also must receive explicit attention, and the therapist must work hard to equip clients with realistic, functional expectations regarding the likely course of their marriage and their moods after the termination of therapy.

## Fading Out the Directive Role of the Therapist

As soon as our clients have mastered the rudiments of communication and problem solving, we attempt to sharply curb the extent of the therapist's directiveness. This results in a decrease in the amount of talking done by the therapist in later sessions as compared with earlier ones. In the end state of therapy, the therapist will typically spend most of the therapy hour listening to the clients recount their week, talk to *each other* (not the therapist) about difficulties or positive experiences they had, and problem solving when necessary. The therapist will guide the interaction by suggesting that the spouses use certain skills or by pinpointing difficulties they are having in communication (e.g., "Why don't you try validating Sharon on this, Jack, before you problem solve?").

Much of the therapist's utterances at the end of therapy are statements of recognition and praise for the clients' handling of situations. The therapist wants to help the clients find a sense of closure about therapy. Most clients cannot afford to nor do they care to remain in therapy until every small difficulty they have is ironed out. The therapist therefore has to begin fading out detailed feedback before the couple is "perfect" in their interaction. This requires ignoring some problems that the therapist judges to be either relatively minor or intractable and selectively praising improvements in their communication or interaction patterns. The therapist also takes his/her cue from the clients in terms of judging whether a difficulty was solved satisfactorily or not. If the clients are satisfied with it, by and large the therapist at the final stage of therapy should simply praise it and leave it alone. Frequently clients may select ways of solving issues that strike the therapist as less than ideal, but the final criterion should be whether or not it works for this couple. For example, when asked about how they stopped arguing about their in-laws, a couple said they were avoiding talking about the issue at all. This is clearly not an ideal solution, but they seemed pleased with it and had no interest in "opening that can of worms." In addition, this couple's differences largely concerned matters of general principle; when concrete issues arose, they could work together within a problem-solving framework. Accordingly, in this case the therapist decided to praise their cooperative decision and move on to other issues.

In the final stage of therapy the therapist will typically ask about how the week went and ask specific questions about what each person did to contribute to the interactions of that week. In this way, the therapist helps reinforce the connection between what the couple is now doing differently and their improved satisfaction. It is common when couples are doing well for them to say, "I don't know, we're just getting along better somehow." The therapist can help them take credit for the difference in their relationship by getting them to see what exactly they are doing differently. This can be accomplished by asking detailed questions about each partner's behavior surrounding the change. For example, "John, it sounds as though you must be doing something different since Gwen is feeling 'more loved.' Does it have anything to do with your calling to tell her you'll be late, like you agreed to do last week?" It is only by identifying their changes that couples become equipped to carry on with their improved relationship after the end of therapy.

The therapist should continually deemphasize his/her importance in the change process of the couple. Especially if therapy has made a marked improvement, couples may tend to attribute almost magical powers to the therapist. It is essential that the therapist avoid the temptation of being "deified." Rather, the therapist's goal at this point in therapy is to empower the clients with the knowledge that it is *their* efforts at change that have made the difference. The mainstay of the therapist's verbal repertoire at the end phase of therapy should be such phrases as, "Why don't you two figure out how you want to handle that problem?," "It sounds like you dealt with that conflict very well," and "Talk to your wife about it, not to me."

## Narrowing the Scope of Therapy

As the therapist is fading out his/her directiveness, the focus of therapy should also be narrowing. Whereas the early and middle phases of therapy presented a variety of techniques to the couple, the final phase should be restricted to practicing those interventions that proved most effective for the particular couple. Again, this narrowing may not be ideal in the eyes of the therapist, who may see that the couple never quite mastered a skill that they could really use. However, the therapist must be realistic about the capacities of the couple and the length of therapy. It is essential that the therapist help the couple to depart therapy with a sense of closure. The final phase of therapy is a time to build on what they have accomplished during the earlier phases, not dwell on what was not accomplished.

For example, one couple we saw had never completely mastered communication skills (i.e., summary, reflection, and validation). However, they had learned how to edit out the extremely negative messages they had previously been using with each other. This, along with an increase in positive time spent together, appeared to have a significant effect in increasing their satisfaction with the marriage and decreasing the wife's depression. Thus, for this couple, these two successful interventions were emphasized and reinforced during the final phase of therapy. Although it may be argued that they should have had a stronger base in communication skills and problem solving in order to maintain gains, it was judged to be more important to consolidate the gains they had already made (and improve their sense of self-efficacy) rather than to struggle in teaching them skills they were having difficulty mastering. For couples such as this one, it may be suggested that more marital work is a possibility in the future if they desire it.

## Trouble-Shooting

The final session with our clients is usually spent highlighting gains and pinpointing possible future trouble spots. We usually ask our clients, "If I were to call you up in a year and things were not going well between you, what would have happened?" Asked in this way, clients can usually say what it is they would have done to let the relationship deteriorate again. The couple can be directed to use their problem-solving skills to examine how best to avoid these probable pitfalls.

When doing trouble-shooting, we focus especially on how the clients can identify problems early, before they are entrenched and before hopelessness sets in. Thus, if a particular couple identified their primary potential problem as neglecting to use the skills they learned in therapy, one solution might be to suggest that they schedule a monthly night out on a regular basis (e.g., the first Friday of each month) and use that night to discuss how they are doing with their relationship. Again, however, the therapist will encourage the couple to be creative and develop a plan that will "fit" them and their lifestyle.

## Problem Solving: Mechanism for Continued Change

The most important skill that a marital therapist can give to clients is to provide them with their own workable mechanisms for changing the relationship when it requires change. Giving clients the ability to solve further difficulties on their own is essential to long-term maintenance of gains in the absence of continuing therapy. We stress that the occurrence of a dysphoric mood or a conflict in the relationship should be viewed as a *cue* to use problem solving or another method of addressing the issue.

For many couples, the best method of addressing new relationship issues or problems as they arise is to use the problem-solving framework they learned in therapy. However, not every couple must use the formal steps of problem solving in order to benefit from the general problem-solving attitude. Again, during the final phase of therapy we try to reinforce whatever level of problem-solving ability the couple has demonstrated previously. The essential thing for couples to take with them at termination is the realization that there are solutions or partial solutions to problems and that it is worthwhile to try to find them. In addition, therapy should have served to normalize the process of change within the marriage. Asking for wanted changes in a spouse's behavior should have become an accepted part of the relationship by the end of therapy. The major focus of the final stage of therapy can be reinforcing this pattern of raising issues for discussion directly and nonaggressively.

## Booster Sessions

It may well be that sustained marital change is something that requires "checkups" periodically. Data from our outcome study indicate that our couples maintained their gains over a 1-year follow-up period. Interestingly, however, several of our couples told us that simply coming in for follow-ups and talking about marital issues was helpful to them as a "reminder" of what they should do. Thus we sometimes schedule regular checkups when a couple leaves therapy. These checkup appointments are used to problem solve about any difficulties the couple has experienced since the last appointment. Sometimes a checkup indicates that further work is necessary or desired, and a series of regular appointments is scheduled. Other times, couples are reluctant to make the effort to come in because they really do not see the need, since the relationship is going well. In these cases the couple is reinforced for their continuing gains and the booster session can be postponed (see also Jacobson, 1989).

## Attitudes and Expectations

Throughout the course of therapy we attempt to provide clients with an understanding of their problems that portrays each partner in a nonblaming manner, in the belief that the way in which each partner views the marriage and the partner is an important determinant of satisfaction. During the final stage of therapy these perceptions of the marriage are often explicitly reviewed. It is sometimes helpful for spouses to notice how their views have changed over the course of therapy. Also, spouses can be encouraged to view the reemergence of a negative view of their relationship as a cue that they should look at what they are doing. This is done in the hope that dissatisfaction can become a cue to begin problem solving or relationship work rather than a sign that "nothing has really changed."

As clients are approaching termination, we also attempt to provide them with functional, realistic expectations regarding the likely course of both their marital satisfaction and their depressive moods. This is done in order to prevent unrealistic expectations from destroying real improvements in functioning. One of the major unrealistic expectations our clients have is that marriage should be blissful. Although many of our clients have experienced significant increases in marital satisfaction, they may undervalue these increases because they compare them to an unrealistic standard of marital bliss. We emphasize with our clients that marriage is not an idyllic state for most people. We also emphasize the inevitable fluctuations in marital satisfaction that occur when a couple leaves therapy. Similarly, the previously depressed spouse is told to expect some fluctuations in mood. We emphasize to our clients that temporary decreases in marital satisfaction and/or increases in depression should be expected. If such fluctuations persist, they should be viewed as cues to action. The only danger in fluctuations in mood or marital satisfaction is that they could be taken to mean "all that work was for nothing . . . we're back where we started." To the contrary, fluctuations are normal and clients must be prepared for them. We emphasize that their therapy has not made them immune to fluctuations; rather it has made them better able to deal with fluctuations and to prevent them from becoming destructive.

## Process Issues in the Final Stage of Therapy

There are several process issues which tend to occur in the final phase of marital therapy with depressed individuals. The therapist should be sensitive to them when approaching termination.

## Fear of Leaving Therapy

The more distressed a couple was before therapy, and the more successful therapy was, the greater is the likelihood that they will experience fear at the thought of termination. It is a common tendency for such couples to attribute more of the change they have experienced to the power of the therapist than to their own efforts, and the therapist must work hard to attribute change to them. The therapist must emphasize the power to change that the couple has demonstrated. Final sessions concentrating on trouble-shooting and problem solving surrounding the issue of relapse should help the fearful clients to see that they can do much to help themselves.

The therapist's stance is also important with regard to decreasing fear on the clients' part. We summarize our stance to our clients at termination as, "I'm here but you don't really need me." That is, the therapist gives the double message of being available to the clients while also telling the clients they probably will not need him/her. The therapist will be aided in promoting this stance if he/she has been successfully fading out influence during the last few therapy sessions. Then the therapist can point to the changes made on the clients' own initiative as evidence that they really can maintain their gains on their own.

Some couples will be sufficiently stressed and frightened by the impending end of therapy that they temporarily regress to their prether-apy level of functioning. By doing so, they "prove" to the therapist that they are not yet ready to leave therapy. Whether or not the therapist suspects that this temporary regression is the result of fear regarding termination, we believe that the clients' needs in terms of further contact should be respected. If a couple appears to be doing well to the therapist but is reluctant to terminate therapy, we feel that the therapist should be sensitive to the couple's obvious message that they are not yet ready to leave. Sometimes this reluctance to leave therapy is due to a hidden issue that has not been previously brought out in therapy. The therapist should ask each spouse, perhaps in a split session, if there are other issues he/she wants to address. For example, we have had clients who were silent about a major sexual difficulty throughout therapy. The issue surfaced only when the therapist questioned their reluctance to terminate despite their success in other problem areas.

## Is That All There Is?

A difficulty some couples encounter late in therapy is that of coming to terms with the limited nature of the gains they have made. While many things about the relationship may have improved, the "new" relationship does not measure up to their hopes or expectations. Especially if a couple was unsure of their commitment but decided to try to do their best in therapy and postpone decisions about dissolving the relationship until the end of therapy, the issue of unmet expectations can be major. Termination of therapy can create a major decision point for such couples.

To deal with unmet expectations, we have found that some split sessions devoted to realistically evaluating the "new" relationship and its ability to satisfy the needs of the two partners can be helpful. Such evaluation must include discussion of realistic expectations, as mentioned above, as well as the plausibility of alternatives to the marriage. Some individuals will decide that the continuation of their marriage is not what they want, and the issue of separation and divorce will need to be addressed.

## Dealing with Separation and Divorce

Separation and divorce are always one possible outcome of marital therapy. People enter couples therapy because they are dissatisfied with their marriages; and given the high rate of divorce in our society, it is inevitable that some of those people decide to divorce. With our population of discordant couples who are also at risk for depression, the issue of the termination of the marriage presents special difficulties. What is the best way to treat a depressed, discordant couple when a decision to divorce has been made?

We consider the therapist's first priority to be the maintenance of the depressed spouse's stability and ability to cope with the divorce or separation. It is important that the therapist discontinue conjoint sessions as soon as it is clear that one partner wants out of the relationship. This is done to protect the depressed or depression-prone spouse from the extreme pain of being in a "marital therapy" session with a spouse who does not want to be married. We find that little or nothing productive can be accomplished in conjoint sessions at this time, and they can be emotionally devastating. Instead, we see both partners individually, if they desire it. The depressed spouse especially should not be abandoned at this time by the therapist. He/she needs support and close monitoring during the first few days and weeks after a decision has been made to separate, since this is a high-risk time for suicide attempts. The therapist should be particularly concerned if the depressed spouse sees the divorce as affecting all areas of his/her life, has poor alternative social relationships, engages in resigned wishful thinking about reestablishing the relationship, or attempts to deny that the decision to divorce represents a real or final decision (Thomssen & Möller, 1988).

In our outcome study, we found that separation during the course of therapy was *not* a negative predictor for improvement in cognitive therapy. In other words, for those women who separated from their husbands during the course of individual cognitive therapy, the improvement in their depression due to the therapy was just as great as in the women whose husbands remained with them. In fact, we have seen that separation can sometimes be a positive force, inducing rapid and dramatic change for the better for those individuals who were in very destructive or discordant relationships. Therefore we recommend that therapists attempt cognitive therapy for depression with a depressed person who has separated from his/her spouse during the course of marital therapy.

## Case Example: Kathy and Sal

Kathy and Sal were a couple in their late 30s who had two small children. Their problems had centered on Kathy's dissatisfaction with Sal's work schedule and lack of help with household work. They both felt overwhelmed by too much work and too little time together. The therapist had pinpointed communication dificulties that centered on a pattern of Kathy's being highly critical and Sal's not talking about problems at all. Earlier work had focused on increasing positive shared time, increasing specific requests for change, and decreasing criticism.

## Session 12

The therapist brought up the issue of termination. Kathy expressed some fear at the thought of leaving therapy. The session focused on a review of the strategies they had found helpful so far—planning enjoyable time together and making it a priority, Kathy's being less critical of and more assertive with Sal, and Sal's willingly talking to Kathy about things that concerned her. The therapist aided them in identifying what they had done during the past week to make it a good week. Their assignment was to continue doing positive joint activities and to continue with a nightly review of their interactions during that day.

## Session 13

When session 13 began, Kathy and Sal were quite upset with each other. They had begun to fight the previous evening about Sal's taking on more responsibility at work, an issue that had been a sore point for years. They had put off discussion of the topic until their session. They were both quite upset and had reverted to their old pattern of Kathy's attacking and Sal's withdrawing and refusing to discuss the issue. The therapist pointed this out and suggested that they use the roles of speaker and listener until they could both express their point of view. This calmed the discussion somewhat. The therapist praised them for their ability to talk civilly about a very disturbing topic. She did not encourage them to try problem solving on this issue, since they had attempted a similar project before and were unable to complete it. Instead, she praised them for their ability to "agree or disagree" in a civilized manner.

## Session 14

The first part of session 14 was spent reviewing the week. Kathy and Sal reported having had a good week, and the therapist asked how they had recovered from their disagreement of last session. Although they seemed to think they had not done anything special, the therapist reminded them that they used to have arguments that lasted for several days. She praised them for not letting the disagreement "poison" the week and for getting back on track with doing positive things for each other. The topic of disciplining their older daughter was then discussed in a collaborative, problem-solving manner, since the daughter had presented some problems during the week. It was suggested that they try out some of the strategies they came up with to discipline her during the following week.

## Session 15

Session 15 was the final regular session for Kathy and Sal. The hour was spent in reviewing successful strategies they had used and in trouble-shooting. Kathy stated her fear that Sal would stop talking to her once they were out of therapy. She was encouraged to state her fear directly to Sal. He suggested that she simply remind him that he was withdrawing in a noncritical way and that he would try his best to respond. Kathy also asked Sal to help monitor her criticism and to tell her when she was becoming too critical. The therapist suggested that they think of a way to continue going out together. They came up with the idea of getting involved in a bowling league that would require them to show up each week. The therapist praised them for this idea. The therapist reminded them that they would be contacted periodically and also reminded them that ups and downs were normal and to be expected.

# 8

## Outcome and Future Directions

Outcome work is a critical component of any therapy that is being recommended for general use (Beach & O'Leary, 1985; Beach & Bauserman, 1990). Outcome research directly addresses an issue of great importance—whether interventions are safe, effective, and applicable to a specifiable population. Likewise, outcome studies force persons proposing new treatments to provide more than a slick sales pitch and claims of phenomenal recoveries to justify the potential usefulness of their approach. However, many other types of research are also important in the initial development of interventions. Prior to formal outcome research, there should be a foundation of clinical observation, basic research, uncontrolled trials, and single case studies that give substantial direction and support to the proposed program of treatment (cf. Agras, Kazdin, & Wilson, 1979). Similarly, once a treatment has been documented as safe and effective for a given population, it seems reasonable to aggressively pursue process work aimed at enhancing overall outcome and specifying population parameters that predict better response (cf. Beach & Bauserman, 1990). In particular, it is likely to be important to carefully investigate the subject, therapy process, and therapist characteristics that are associated with the greatest gain in therapy. Accordingly, studies aimed at better understanding nonresponders to treatment or noncompliance with treatment should have a high priority once effectiveness has been established for a specifiable population. Only after process work and the refinement of the treatment program does comparison with other approaches become informative. At this stage of development, the comparison of two equally well developed approaches to treatment can have direct implications for clinical decision making (cf. Agras et al., 1979). Given the overall framework for outcome research presented above, we believe that current outcome work on marital therapy for co-occurring marital discord and depression should be viewed as providing a preliminary estimate of the effectiveness of this program and an initial sketch of the optimal form this therapy may ultimately take. Sufficient process work has not yet been done to determine how good this intervention can ultimately be or how it might be revised to achieve optimal effectiveness. Likewise, the exact population parameters indicative of optimal response are only partially known. We would envision future work aimed at identifying obstacles to change and mediators of outcome as necessary before a "second generation" of outcome studies could begin to tell us just how far a marital approach to depression can take us. However, despite our view that comparison outcome studies are premature, some comparison of new approaches with established approaches can help researchers and therapists alike characterize the new approach as "promising" if it shows an advantage over an established intervention, or as "disappointing" if it does not. In the case of marital therapy for the maritally discordant and depressed, the obvious advantage over somatic or individual approaches for which one might look is superior improvement in marital satisfaction with equal improvement in level of depression.

## Review of Initial Uncontrolled Observations

Our own uncontrolled observations took place in the context of the University Marital Therapy Clinic at Stony Brook, New York. It was a commonplace observation in this setting that as marital discord was resolved through directive, short-term marital interventions, reports of problems with regard to depression and anxiety were often dramatically reduced without, or with minimal, direct intervention. Furthermore, many of the depressed persons being seen in the marital clinic appeared to their therapists to be as depressed as persons seeking individual therapy for depression. Thus the observation that these "depressed spouses" were improving in marital therapy suggested that in some manner, at least within this population of overtly maritally discordant couples, marital therapy was "curing" depression (see Beach & Nelson, 1990).

It should be noted that these clinical observations were compelling and striking. We were quite sure that many couples presenting for marital therapy met standard clinical criteria for depression. Indeed, as we examined these couples more closely we found that over 50% of couples presenting for marital therapy had at least one spouse scoring in the depressed range on the Beck Depression Inventory (Beach et al., 1985). In addition, there were reports in the literature that couples with more depressive symptoms improved more with regard to marital satisfaction than other couples presenting for marital therapy (Jacobson, Follette, &

Pagel, 1986). There were also case reports from other laboratories and clinics examining the possible effectiveness of marital therapy with depressed patients. For example, Lewinsohn had proposed relatively early on that feedback to spouses about their interactive behavior could help decrease depression (Lewinsohn, 1974; Lewinsohn & Atwood, 1969; Lewinsohn & Shaffer, 1971). Indeed, given the salience of the marital environment as a source of reinforcement and punishment for spouses, Lewinsohn's (1974) theoretical perspective provided an early and natural impetus to examine the possible effectiveness of maritally focused interventions. Likewise, Jacobson and Margolin (1979) noted that marital therapy "is the recommended treatment mode when depressive behaviors are elicited or maintained by relationship processes" (p. 311). In a case report they discussed the need to increase pleasant events and communication skills. Thus this case report provided an early example of the possible effectiveness of a marital therapy approach similar to the one in use at the University Marital Therapy Clinic at Stony Brook.

## Review of Early Outcome and Analogue Work on Effects of Marital Therapy for Depression

Through a confluence of clinical observation, initial single-subject studies, and theoretical support for the likely value of marital interventions in depression, a number of researchers were sufficiently encouraged to attempt randomized trials in which one condition could be viewed as largely "marital" in focus. For example, McLean, Ogston, and Grauer (1973) demonstrated the superiority of a focused behavioral marital intervention over alternative treatments available in the community (e.g., medication, group therapy, individual therapy, combinations of the former) for a population of apparently discordant, depressed patients. The authors did not use standard measures of marital satisfaction and did not select for maritally discordant couples. However, they reported the presence of marital disputes in all couples. The authors also did not assess depressive symptoms per se. However, they were able to show significant improvement in depressed mood on the Depression Adjective Checklist (Lubin, 1965), improvement on target behaviors, and improvement on positiveness of communication for the group treated with a form of marital therapy. Thus, while diagnostic questions, measurement issues, and the nonstandard nature of the marital intervention limit the interpretability of the study, it still must be viewed as a pioneering study suggesting the potential for marital therapy in the treatment of depression.

Another early controlled study of marital therapy for diagnosed depression was reported by Friedman (1975). While this study is often cited as evidence of the effectiveness of marital therapy for depression, the effects demonstrated were actually quite modest. When analyses using only "completers" of therapy were reported, marital therapy actually looked nonsignificantly worse than placebo–minimal contact on the global rating of therapy outcome. Even when the more favorable analysis—which included dropouts across all conditions—was reported, marital therapy displayed a rather weak effect on depressive symptoms and on relationship behavior. Indeed, it is probably only the even more striking weakness displayed by the antidepressant medication group that allowed the author to say anything positive about marital therapy for depression. It is worth noting, however, that no effort was made in this study to separate maritally discordant from nondiscordant couples. Our expectation is that this should have resulted in the inclusion of a large group of probable nonresponders in the marital therapy condition (cf. Whisman et al., 1988). In addition, the group was very heterogeneous with regard to diagnoses (which were pre-DSM-III diagnoses in any case). The heterogeneity with regard to Axis I and Axis II diagnoses could also increase variability in response to treatment (see Chapter 4). Thus, while only minimally positive in outcome, the marital therapy study reported by Friedman (1975) was encouraging of further investigation of marital therapy for depression.

Another study which was encouraging of a marital approach to the treatment of psychiatric disorders, including depression, was reported by Hafner, Badenoch, Fisher, and Swift (1983). In this study, patients with a wide variety of psychiatric disorders of a severe and persisting nature were treated with either a marital or an individual approach to therapy. Psychiatric symptoms in general were improved somewhat more by the marital interventions than by the individual approaches. However, it is particularly interesting that individual therapy was found to be associated with improvement in symptomatic status, even while producing an overall increase in marital problems, and increased depression for both partners at 3-month follow-up. Thus, while not a study of a particular diagnostic category, the results once again suggest the promise of a marital approach to the treatment of depression and the likely ineffectiveness of individual approaches in resolving marital disputes.

These early studies, while encouraging, had various limitations that precluded their being taken as a solid foundation for recommending marital therapy as we conducted it for the treatment of depressed, discordant couples. The early studies typically indicated that they had employed one form or another of nonstandard or very loosely specified interventions. Likewise, it was unclear from these studies that individuals meeting current diagnostic criteria for major depressive episode, unipolar type, could benefit from marital approaches.

Accordingly, our first step beyond simple clinical observation was to pilot the use of marital therapy for couples in which one member was depressed (i.e., met DSM-III criteria for either unipolar depression, single episode, or unipolar depression, recurrent). The primary purpose of the study was to determine whether marital therapy, as it was practiced at the University Marital Therapy Clinic at Stony Brook, could be successfully applied to a population suffering from both depression and marital discord. A secondary purpose was to determine whether individual cognitive therapy could also be successful in reducing depressive symptoms in this population, since persons suffering from both marital discord and depression had been reported to be difficult to treat successfully (cf. Rounsaville et al., 1979a, 1979b).

## An Initial Pilot Study

Only wives who (1) met criteria for major affective disorder, unipolar type (i.e., DSM-III 296.2 or DSM-III 296.3) with no psychotic features, (2) presented marital discord as a major problem, and (3) agreed to random assignment to behavioral marital therapy, individual cognitive therapy, or a waiting list control group (in which some phone consultation could be requested) were included in the study (Beach & O'Leary, 1986). Of the eight couples meeting these criteria, three were assigned to individual cognitive therapy, three to behavioral marital therapy, and two to a waiting list control condition.

Spouses ranged in age from 23 to 50, with the modal couple being in their early 30s. Education level attained ranged from elementary school to graduate school, with the modal level being a high school graduate. Income ranged from $13,000 per year to $60,000 per year, with the modal couple having a combined family income of approximately $25,000. The average number of years married was 14, with a range from 5 to 28.

The therapists employed in the study were graduate students (two males, one female) enrolled in the Ph.D. program at the State University of New York at Stony Brook. Two of the therapists were married. All therapists received training in cognitive therapy (28 hours) and behavioral marital therapy (30 hours) beyond the normal training requirements of the clinical psychology program. Each therapist saw one individual cognitive therapy and one conjoint behavioral marital therapy case. Thus therapist effects were distributed equally across the two therapy conditions.

The primary measures used to assess gains in therapy were the Dyadic Adjustment Scale (DAS; Spanier, 1976), a refinement and extension of the Locke–Wallace Marital Adjustment Scale (Locke & Wallace,

1959), and the Beck Depression Inventory (BDI; Beck et al., 1979), a widely used measure of depressive symptomatology consisting of 21 items, each corresponding to a specific category of symptoms and attitudes (Beck et al., 1988).

## Procedure

Patients meeting preliminary screening requirements met with a trained psychologist who administered the Schedule for Affective Disorders and Schizophrenia (SADS-C; Endicott & Spitzer, 1978). Diagnoses were made on the basis of this interview, but in accordance with DSM-III diagnostic criteria. Patients and spouses were also asked to complete the standard assessment battery at this time. During a separate interview, spouses were asked about their marital relationship. Couples selected for participation in the study were assigned to one of three conditions.

### THERAPY CONDITIONS

Behavioral marital therapy (BMT) focused on increasing positive instrumental behaviors, improving problem-solving and communication skills, setting reasonable expectations of spouses, and gaining insight into the reasons for the development of marital discord. The techniques outlined in Chapters 5 through 7 played a prominent role in this form of therapy.

Cognitive therapy (CT) was also used. This procedure assumes that an individual's affect and behavior are largely determined by the way in which he/she structures the world. The therapeutic techniques employed are designed to identify, reality test, and correct distorted conceptualizations and the dysfunctional schemata underlying them. Techniques used included monitoring automatic thoughts, generating alternative interpretations of events, and graded task assignments. Cognitive therapy as used in this study followed the procedures outlined by Beck and colleagues (1979).

### TREATMENT ON DEMAND (TOD)

Couples in this condition were told that they were on a treatment waiting list but that they could request therapeutic consultation. Consultation was to focus on immediate crisis intervention and was not to include either cognitive or marital interventions. However, as neither couple in this condition requested crisis work, these couples received the same assessments given the other couples, but no therapy.

All couples were assessed using the BDI and the DAS following sessions 2, 4, 6, 8, 10, 12, and 14 or during the corresponding weeks in the waiting list condition. These reports allowed us to examine the course of change in marital adjustment and in level of depressive symptomatology. Following their last session, couples returned to the clinic to complete an assessment battery containing the same forms completed at pretherapy. They were also interviewed about their reactions to therapy and about their perceptions of the changes that had occurred as a result of therapy. This interview procedure was repeated at a 3-month follow-up.

## Results

Reduction in level of depression was marked for wives in both treated groups. Wives receiving BMT began therapy with BDI scores of 25, 17, and 15 and ended therapy with BDI scores of 0, 7, and 2, respectively. Similarly, wives in CT began therapy with BDI scores of 14, 19, and 30, and *all* ended therapy with BDI scores of 0. All wives in both conditions reported to interviewers that they were no longer depressed at the end of therapy and at 3-month follow-up. When the biweekly means for improvement in BDI for each group were plotted and compared using a Wilcoxon signed-ranks test, there was no significant difference in amount of change in depression over the course of therapy or at 3-month follow-up between wives receiving CT and those receiving BMT. Comparisons with the wives in the waiting-list condition suggested that both CT and BMT were successful in alleviating depression in this sample relative to any spontaneously occurring remission. Both BMT [$T(8) = 0$, $p < .01$] and CT couples [$T(8) = 0$, $p < .01$] differed from those on the waiting list on BDI change.

Wives receiving BMT showed clear increases in level of satisfaction, with pretherapy DAS scores of 66, 98, and 78 and posttherapy scores of 96, 114, and 100, respectively. Wives receiving CT showed improvement as well, with initial scores of 97, 110, and 109 and posttherapy scores of 116, 128, and 111, respectively. However, when the biweekly means for marital improvement and therapy were plotted for both treated groups, improvement over the course of therapy and at 3-month follow-up was found to be significantly greater with BMT than with CT [$T(7) = 1$, $p < .05$]. Overall, the wives in BMT showed more rapid and greater gains in marital functioning during the course of therapy and at 3-month follow-up than did wives receiving CT. Consideration of spouses' report of change in marital satisfaction over the course of therapy corroborates the impression that BMT provided more rapid and greater gains in marital functioning in this sample. The pattern of change reported by husbands mirrors the report of wives. BMT was significantly better than being on the waiting list in producing gains in marital satisfaction [$T(5) = 0$, $p < .05$] and was also significantly better than CT [$T(7) = 0$, $p < .01$].

Importantly, all participants receiving either individual CT or BMT rated the program as moderately to extremely helpful; all treated subjects also indicated that they would recommend the program to a friend.

Both CT and BMT emerged from this initial pilot study as reasonable approaches to working with women who are simultaneously suffering both depression and marital discord. The results tended to confirm our initial clinical impression that, with a carefully defined population, behavioral marital therapy could be as effective in reducing depressive symptomatology as standard and accepted interventions for depression. In addition, the results supported our hypothesis that marital therapy could do better than cognitive therapy in improving the marital environment of depressed patients in discordant marital relationships. However, cognitive therapy emerged as a very potent and reasonable intervention for this population as well, particularly with regard to the reduction of depressive symptomatology.

## A Larger-Scale Outcome Study

Encouraged by these initial results, we began a somewhat larger-scale outcome study in order to answer more definitively the question of the potential utility of marital therapy as a treatment modality for depression (O'Leary & Beach, 1990). Thirty-six couples were randomly assigned to either individual CT, conjoint BMT, or a 15-week waiting-list condition. Interestingly, as we recruited larger numbers of subjects we found increasing numbers of subjects receiving dysthymia diagnoses or other diagnoses in addition to the diagnosis of major depressive episode. Indeed, approximately half of the wives in our second study received an additional Axis I diagnosis in addition to major depression. Three wives who did not receive a diagnosis of major depressive episode were diagnosed as being dysthymic. Persons receiving medication for depression or related symptoms were not included in the study, nor were persons with active suicidal ideation. As in the pilot study, wives had to have an initial BDI score greater than or equal to 14. In addition, both partners had to score in the maritally discordant range of the DAS.

The average age of the subjects involved in the study was 42. The average number of children per family was 2.5, and the average educational level of the female subjects was 14 years. There were three therapists who provided both CT and BMT. The therapists were trained in marital therapy and cognitive therapy by clinical experts in the field (W. Edward Craighead, Duke University, and Norman Epstein, University of Maryland, cognitive therapy; Donald H. Baucom, University of North Carolina, and K. Daniel O'Leary, State University of New York at Stony Brook, marital therapy). In addition, the recognized experts provided periodic clinical consultation to the therapists.

## Results Posttherapy

### DEPRESSION

Both BMT and CT were effective in reducing depressive symptomatology. The three groups were significantly different at posttreatment $[F(2,33) = 6.46, p = .004]$, and both the BMT and CT subjects respectively had significantly lower depression scores than the waiting-list control subjects $[F(1,22) = 11.67, p = .017; F(1,21) = 5.23, p < .032]$. The marital therapy and individual therapy groups did not have significantly different depression scores at posttherapy $[F(1,22) = 1.23, p = .278]$.

### MARITAL SATISFACTION

An analysis of variance (ANOVA) indicated that there were significant differences in marital satisfaction across the three groups at posttherapy $[F(2,33) = 5.13, p < .012]$. The marital therapy subjects had significantly higher marital satisfaction scores at posttherapy than the cognitive therapy subjects $[F(1,22) = 8.65, p = .008]$ and the waiting-list control subjects $[F(1,22) = 7.65, p = .011]$. However, the individual therapy subjects did not differ from the waiting-list control subjects $[F(1,22) = 0.42, p = .526]$.

## 1-Year Follow-Up

ANOVAs indicated that the marital therapy group did not have lower depression scores than the cognitive therapy group at follow-up $[F(1,22) = 1.84, p = .188]$, but as reflected in Figures 8-1 and 8-2, the marital therapy group had significantly higher marital satisfaction scores at follow-up than the CT group $[F(1,22) = 5.41, p = .030]$.

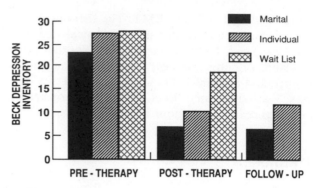

FIGURE 8-1. Changes in depression across treatment and waiting-list groups.

## Clinically Significant Improvement

Another way to assess the efficacy of treatment is to determine the number of individuals who reached a generally accepted criterion of not being clinically depressed and/or who made significant changes on critical dependent measures during therapy. At posttherapy, 67% of the individual therapy subjects and 83% of the marital therapy subjects no longer met our initial inclusion criteria for being in an episode of depression (BDI ≤ 14). At posttherapy, 25% of the individual therapy subjects and 83% of the marital therapy subjects had at least 15-point pre–post increases in their marital satisfaction scores. The same general pattern of results held at follow-up; that is, both the decreases in depression and the increases in marital satisfaction were maintained 1 year following treatment.

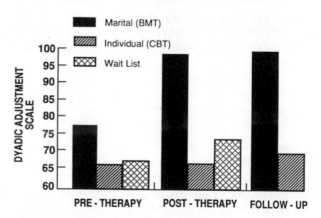

FIGURE 8-2. Changes in marital adjustment across treatment and waiting-list groups.

Again, the results of this larger study are compelling. Marital therapy is a safe and effective intervention for a specifiable population; that is, for mildly to moderately depressed women in relationships where marital discord is overt and recognized. For this population, marital therapy may well be the therapy of choice. It appears to be as effective as more widely used individual interventions and to have additional benefits with regard to improvement in the marital relationship. The beneficial effects of marital therapy do not appear to be transitory, and the satisfaction expressed by consumers was considerable. Couples falling in the category described above appeared to be eager for marital therapy and often expressed the belief that marital therapy was exactly the therapy they needed.

## Related Ongoing Outcome Work

A large-scale investigation of marital therapy for depression involving both explicitly discordant and nondiscordant, depressed couples is currently ongoing (Whisman et al., 1988). In this study, depressed women who were in intact marriages, reporting a range of marital satisfaction, were randomly assigned to marital therapy, cognitive therapy alone, or a combination of cognitive and marital therapy. The authors have reported effects of BMT similar to those obtained by O'Leary and Beach (1990) *only* for the most maritally discordant portion of their depressed population (i.e., both spouses scored $\leq 100$ on the DAS). Indeed, for the *less discordant couples*, cognitive therapy was found to produce beneficial effects, with marital therapy showing no positive benefit. Thus, in line with our initial speculation, it appears that marital approaches to depression may be most appropriate for the explicitly discordant, depressed group and may be inappropriate in cases where depression is not associated with overt discord.

Preliminary evidence is also available from work being done on the inclusion of a spouse in interpersonal psychotherapy for depression (IPT; Foley, Rounsaville, Weissman, Sholomskas, & Chevron, in press; Weissman, 1988). Data currently available indicate that the inclusion of the spouse in those cases where marital disputes are present is at least as effective as individual IPT in alleviating symptoms of depression, and somewhat more effective at improving marital quality. This work was conducted with an inpatient population with considerably more severe depressive symptomatology than was present in either our own outcome work or that conducted by Whisman and colleagues (1988). Thus, by finding a similar pattern of results, this work (Weissman, 1988) suggests the potential for marital therapy to play a useful role as an adjunct to pharmacological interventions when the initial level of depression is moderate to severe.

As can be seen, the considerable possibilities of marital intervention in the treatment of depression have sparked interest among researchers. In addition, the results to date suggest that marital interventions, particularly marital interventions such as those outlined in this book, have great potential as both primary and adjunctive treatments for ongoing depressive episodes. However, it is also clear that the investigations to date represent only preliminary approaches to optimal marital therapy for depression. Process work aimed at clarifying subject characteristics, therapist characteristics, and process characteristics related to less than optimal outcome are only now beginning. Likewise, the issue of long-term maintenance of therapeutic gain has not yet been investigated. Thus we do not yet know either how good marital therapy can ultimately be or how long it will retain its superiority to other forms of treatment for the discordant, depressed couple. These areas must remain high-priority ones for research and clinical observation.

## Future Directions

Several issues of primary importance for future research on the clinical application of marital therapy to the treatment of depression are alluded to in the review of research above. First, there is the issue of maintenance of gains within the realms of both marital discord and depressive symptomatology. It is a commonplace observation that depression is a recurring problem. Often resolution of a particular episode is not particularly difficult, and in most cases depression will be a self-limiting problem even in the absence of treatment. Of more importance may be the ability of a treatment to provide some prophylaxis against future episodes. While there are strong theoretical grounds for believing that a marital relationsip improved via marital therapy should enhance resistance to relapse of depression (Jacobson, 1985), this has yet to be empirically demonstrated. Accordingly, long-term follow-up of successfully treated patients should be a high priority for future clinical investigation. Indeed, a better understanding of relapse and ways to prevent relapse is important for basic work in the area of marital therapy as well as in the application of marital therapy to the treatment of depression (Beach & Bauserman, 1990). While our own work suggests that the effects of marital therapy for depression show good maintenance for 1 year, there is reason to believe that maintenance for marital therapy in general may be poorer at latencies longer than 1 year (Jacobson, Schmaling, & Holtzworth-Munroe,

1987). Thus particular attention should be given in the future to strategies for enhancing maintenance of gains over longer periods of time.

There is also the issue of the limits of applicability of marital therapy to a depressed population. It is simply unclear at present exactly which depressed patients are likely to be most helped by a marital therapy approach. At the same time, it is unclear whether or not marital therapy should be seen as being more generally applicable to many forms of psychiatric dysfunction (Badenoch, Fisher, Hafner, & Swift, 1984; Jacobson, Holtzworth-Munroe, & Schmaling, 1989). It may be that marital interventions will prove applicable for agoraphobia, alcohol and drug problems, and a variety of other psychiatric and behavioral difficulties. It is unclear as well whether the marital discord model elaborated in this book will help illuminate points of intervention for these psychiatric disorders or whether substantially different marital processes will be implicated. While we attempted to provide some suggestions in Chapter 4 regarding the subpopulations of depressed individuals most likely to respond to marital therapy, this too must be considered an area in need of considerable work and clarification.

Where does the current state of knowledge leave the clinician interested in applying marital therapy to the treatment of depression? For the time being, it appears safe to assume that marital therapy can be an effective tool in working with many discordant, depressed patients. Marital therapy appears likely to emerge as the treatment of choice for individuals meeting criteria for unipolar depression who are both displaying mild to moderate depressive symptomatology and complaining of prominent symptoms of marital discord. Likewise, in a population of couples presenting for marital therapy at a marital therapy clinic or in private practice, there are likely to be many couples with a depressed spouse for whom a marital discord model of depression is applicable and illuminating. Through continued clinical observation, creativity, and basic as well as applied research, it appears that attention to marital interventions in the treatment of co-occurring marital discord and depression will substantially advance the effectiveness of our clinical work with this large and difficult population. Clearly, there is a place and a need for marital interventions in the treatment of depression.

# APPENDIX

# Marital Therapy Scale

Therapist _____

Patient _____

Rater _____

Session(s) _____

Date of rating _____

## Therapist Technical Marital Therapy Skills

1. a. Therapist skill in addressing the need for a rapid end to high-intensity negative behavior toward the spouse (e.g., shouting, tantrums, hitting, character assassination, etc.; NA if not required, 0 if not displayed even though required)

   0—

   6—

   b. Outcome with this couple, this session

   | No impact | Clear improvement | | | "Magic moment" |
   |:---:|:---:|:---:|:---:|:---:|
   | 0 | 2 | 4 | 5 | 6 | 8 |

2. a. Therapist skill in presenting a compelling rationale for increasing caring gestures (NA if not required, 0 if required but not displayed)

   0—

   6—

b. Outcome with this couple, this session

No impact     Clear improvement     "Magic moment"
    0         2     4     5     6          8

3. a. Therapist skill in increasing positive joint activities
      0—
      6—
   b. Outcome with this couple, this session

No impact     Clear improvement     "Magic moment"
    0         2     4     5     6          8

4. a. Therapist skill in increasing positive tracking of spouse behavior and compliments
      0—
      6—
   b. Outcome with this couple, this session

No impact     Clear improvement     "Magic moment"
    0         2     4     5     6          8

5. a. Therapist ability to set positive expectations for therapeutic gains
      0—
      6—
   b. Outcome with this couple, this session

No impact     Clear improvement     "Magic moment"
    0         2     4     5     6          8

6. a. Therapist ability to identify and help the couple challenge spousal misperceptions
      0—
      6—
   b. Outcome with this couple, this session

No impact     Clear improvement     "Magic moment"
    0         2     4     5     6          8

7. a. Therapist skill in finding positive implications or connotations of symptomatic or problematic behaviors

0—

6—

   b. Outcome with this couple, this session

| No impact | Clear improvement | | | "Magic moment" |
|---|---|---|---|---|
| 0 | 2 | 4 | 5 | 6 | 8 |

8. a. Therapist skill in helping clients express underlying positive feelings behind complaints (e.g., "I was angry when you were late getting home because I missed you").

0—

6—

   b. Outcome with this couple, this session

| No impact | Clear improvement | | | "Magic moment" |
|---|---|---|---|---|
| 0 | 2 | 4 | 5 | 6 | 8 |

9. a. Therapist skill in providing an alternative framework for clients for understanding their problems in a less accusatory or more benign way

0—

6—

   b. Outcome with this couple, this session

| No impact | Clear improvement | | | "Magic moment" |
|---|---|---|---|---|
| 0 | 2 | 4 | 5 | 6 | 8 |

10. a. Therapist skill in identifying problematic attributions for spouse's behavior and intervening to alter them

0—

6—

   b. Outcome with this couple, this session

| No impact | Clear improvement | | | "Magic moment" |
|---|---|---|---|---|
| 0 | 2 | 4 | 5 | 6 | 8 |

11. a. Therapist skill in identifying implicit "shoulds" in each spouse's stance toward the intervening to soften the sharply defined positions each spouse is taking

    0—

    6—

    b. Outcome with this couple, this session

    | No impact | | Clear improvement | | | "Magic moment" |
    |---|---|---|---|---|---|
    | 0 | 2 | 4 | 5 | 6 | 8 |

12. a. Therapist skill in identifying intent–impact discrepancies and helping clarify the miscommunication

    0—

    6—

    b. Outcome with this couple, this session

    | No impact | | Clear improvement | | | "Magic moment" |
    |---|---|---|---|---|---|
    | 0 | 2 | 4 | 5 | 6 | 8 |

13. a. Therapist skill in providing feedback and redirection regarding the use of negative communication strategies (e.g., cross-complaining, fault finding, use of guilt, giving ultimatums, threatening)

    0—

    6—

    b. Outcome with this couple, this session

    | No impact | | Clear improvement | | | "Magic moment" |
    |---|---|---|---|---|---|
    | 0 | 2 | 4 | 5 | 6 | 8 |

14. a. Therapist skill in teaching attending behavior (e.g., open posture, leaning forward, nodding, visual attending)

    0—

    6—

    b. Outcome with this couple, this session

    | No impact | | Clear improvement | | | "Magic moment" |
    |---|---|---|---|---|---|
    | 0 | 2 | 4 | 5 | 6 | 8 |

15. a. Therapist skill in identifying and correcting problems in nonverbal communication (e.g., voice tone, arousal, gestures)

    0—

    6—

  b. Outcome with this couple, this session

     No impact     Clear improvement     "Magic moment"
        0      2      4      5      6        8

16. a. Therapist skill in teaching reflective listening skills (e.g., skill in role-playing behavior, skill in helping the couple paraphrase)

    0—

    6—

  b. Outcome with this couple, this session

     No impact     Clear improvement     "Magic moment"
        0      2      4      5      6        8

17. a. Therapist skill in teaching supportive comunication (e.g., attending, reflecting, and validating without rushing in to do problem solving)

    0—

    6—

  b. Outcome with this couple, this session

     No impact     Clear improvement     "Magic moment"
        0      2      4      5      6        8

18. a. Therapist skill in teaching validation of partner's position

    0—

    6—

  b. Outcome with this couple, this session

     No impact     Clear improvement     "Magic moment"
        0      2      4      5      6        8

19. a. Therapist skill in teaching good nondefensive question-asking behavior in the context of effective listening

    0—

    6—

   b. Outcome with this couple, this session

     No impact    Clear improvement    "Magic moment"
       0    2    4    5    6    8

20. a. Therapist skill in teaching "sender" skills (e.g., appropriate length, appropriate editing, appropriate clarity)
     0—
     6—
   b. Outcome with this couple, this session

     No impact    Clear improvement    "Magic moment"
       0    2    4    5    6    8

21. a. Therapist skill in teaching affective expression skills ("I-statements," requests, compliments)
     0—
     6—
   b. Outcome with this couple, this session

     No impact    Clear improvement    "Magic moment"
       0    2    4    5    6    8

22. a. Therapist skill in helping the couple create or reestablish routines that create the opportunity for self-disclosure and increased cohesive behavior
     0—
     6—
   b. Outcome with this couple, this session

     No impact    Clear improvement    "Magic moment"
       0    2    4    5    6    8

23. a. Therapist skill in increasing frequency of genuine positive self-disclosure for the couple
     0—
     6—
   b. Outcome with this couple, this session

     No impact    Clear improvement    "Magic moment"
       0    2    4    5    6    8

24. a. Therapist skill in establishing a problem-solving set during problem-solving training and application (e.g., telling the couple to focus on win–win solutions, establishing the overriding goal of strengthening the couple, having the couple recognize the inherently cooperative nature of joint problem solving)

    0—

    6—

    b. Outcome with this couple, this session

    | No impact | | Clear improvement | | | "Magic moment" |
    |---|---|---|---|---|---|
    | 0 | 2 | 4 | 5 | 6 | 8 |

25. a. Therapist skill in selecting a problem appropriate to the level of the clients

    0—

    6—

    b. Outcome with this couple, this session

    | No impact | | Clear improvement | | | "Magic moment" |
    |---|---|---|---|---|---|
    | 0 | 2 | 4 | 5 | 6 | 8 |

26. a. Therapist skill in teaching problem definition

    0—

    6—

    b. Outcome with this couple, this session

    | No impact | | Clear improvement | | | "Magic moment" |
    |---|---|---|---|---|---|
    | 0 | 2 | 4 | 5 | 6 | 8 |

27. a. Therapist skill in teaching the couple to generate alternatives (e.g., keeping on track, no censoring)

    0—

    6—

    b. Outcome with this couple, this session

    | No impact | | Clear improvement | | | "Magic moment" |
    |---|---|---|---|---|---|
    | 0 | 2 | 4 | 5 | 6 | 8 |

28. a. Therapist skill in teaching the couple to evaluate and select an alternative

    0—

    6—

b. Outcome with this couple, this session

No impact      Clear improvement      "Magic moment"
0      2      4      5      6      8

29. a. Therapist skill in teaching the couple to implement, evaluate, and redis-
cuss the solution chosen
0—
6—
b. Outcome with this couple, this session

No impact      Clear improvement      "Magic moment"
0      2      4      5      6      8

30. a. Therapist skill in encouraging time apart doing individual activities in the
context of decreasing one spouse's dependence
0—
6—
b. Outcome with this couple, this session

No impact      Clear improvement      "Magic moment"
0      2      4      5      6      8

## Therapist General Therapy Skills

1. Therapist skill in setting an agenda, keeping to an agenda, and structuring
therapy time
0—
6—

2. Therapist skill in allowing clients' agenda to guide the material covered in the
session
0—
6—

3. Therapist skill in pacing the session and using time efficiently
0—
6—

4. Therapist skill in listening for relevant client material that is not stated directly by the clients (and checking this out with the clients)
   0—
   6—

5. Therapist skill in handling incidents that throw therapy temporarily off-track (without punitive or "cool" responses toward the dyad)
   0—
   6—

6. Therapist skill in assigning homework in a way that makes it meaningful to the clients
   0—
   6—

7. Therapist skill in reviewing homework
   0—
   6—

8. Therapist skill in reinforcing changes and acting as a cheerleader for the relationship
   0—
   6—

9. Therapist warmth
   0—
   6—

10. Therapist ability to use humor effectively
    0—
    6—

11. Therapist ability to form and maintain a strong "dual" therapeutic alliance
    0—
    6—

12. Therapist ability to convince the couple that the issues being addressed are important and relevant to their concerns
    0—
    6—

13. Therapist ability to pick up main themes of the clients' problems
    0—
    6—

14. Therapist ability to avoid excessive focus on negative feelings in the relationship and to maintain a focus on the couple's commitment to change and their gains
    0—
    6—

15. Therapist ability to remain nonjudgmental
    0—
    6—

16. Therapist skill in presenting didactic material in an interesting manner
    0—
    6—

17. Therapist skill in minimizing lecturing and maximizing couple involvement
    0—
    6—

18. Therapist skill in handling outbursts and venting during the therapy session
    0—
    6— .

## Additional Considerations

1. a. Did any special problems arise during the session?
      Briefly describe _____
      _____
      _____

   b. Therapist skill in handling these special problems
      0—
      6—

2. How would you rate the therapist overall in this session in terms of doing good marital therapy?

   | 0 | 1 | 2 | 3 | 4 | 5 | 6 |
   |---|---|---|---|---|---|---|
   | Poor | Barely adequate | Mediocre | Satisfactory | Good | Very good | Excellent |

3. a. How difficult did you feel this client was to work with?
      0—Very receptive (easy)
      6—Extremely difficult
   b. Briefly describe client or couple characteristics contributing to their being
      difficult _____
      _____
      _____

      General comments and suggestions for therapist's improvement _____
      _____
      _____

# References

Abplanap, J. M., Donnelly, A. F., & Rose, R. M. (1979). Psychoendocrinology of the menstrual cycle: I. Enjoyment of daily activities and moods. *Psychosomatic Medicine, 41*, 587–604.

Abramson, L. Y., Metalsky, G. I., & Alloy, L. B. (1989). Hopelessness depression: A theory-based subtype of depression. *Psychological Review, 96*, 358–372.

Abramson, L. Y., Seligman, M. E. P., & Teasdale, J. (1978). Learned helplessness in humans: Critique and reformulation. *Journal of Abnormal Psychology, 87*, 49–74.

Agras, W. S., Kazdin, A. E., & Wilson, G. T. (1979). *Behavior therapy: Toward an applied clinical science.* San Francisco: Freeman.

Akiskal, H. S. (1979). A biobehavioral approach to depression. In R. A. Depue (Ed.), *The psychobiology of the depressive disorders: Implications for the effects of stress.* New York: Academic.

Allen, M. G. (1976). Twin studies of affective illness. *Archives of General Psychiatry, 33*, 1476–1478.

Altman, I., & Taylor, D. A. (1973). *Social penetration: The development of interpersonal relationships.* New York: Holt, Rinehart & Winston.

American Psychiatric Association. (1980). *Diagnostic and statistical manual of mental disorders* (3rd ed.). Washington, DC: Author.

American Psychiatric Association. (1987). *Diagnostic and statistical manual of mental disorders* (3rd ed.—rev.). Washington, DC: Author.

Andreasen, N. C. (1984). *The broken brain: The biological revolution in psychiatry.* New York: Harper & Row.

Andreasen, N. C., Rice, J., Endicott, J., Coryell, W., Grove, W. M., & Reich, T. (1987). Familial rates of affective disorder. *Archives of General Psychiatry, 44*, 461–469.

Arana, G. W., Baldessarini, R. J., & Ornsteen, M. (1985). The dexamethasone suppression test for diagnosis and prognosis in psychiatry: Commentary and review. *Archives of General Psychiatry, 42*, 1193–1204.

Arias, I., & O'Leary, K. D. (1988). Cognitive-behavioral treatment of physical aggression in marriage. In N. Epstein, S. Schlesinger, & W. Dryden (Eds.), *Cognitive-behavioral therapy with families.* New York: Brunner/Mazel.

Arieti, S. & Bemporad, J. (1978). *Severe and mild depression: The psychotherapeutic approach.* New York: Basic Books.

Arkowitz, H., Holliday, S., & Hutter, M. (1982, November). *Depressed women and their husbands: A study of marital interaction and adjustment.* Paper presented at the annual meeting of the Association for Advancement of Behavior Therapy, Los Angeles.

Badenoch, A., Fisher, J., Hafner, R. J., & Swift, H. (1984). Predicting the outcome of spouse-aided therapy for persisting psychiatric disorders. *American Journal of Family Therapy, 12*, 59-71.

Baldessarini, R. J. (1988). Update on recent advances in antidepressant pharmacology and pharmacotherapy. In F. Flach (Ed.), *Psychobiology and psychopharmacology.* New York: Norton.

Bandura, A. (1986). *Social foundations of thought and action: A social cognitive theory.* Englewood Cliffs, NJ: Prentice-Hall.

Barlow, D. H. (1980). Behavior therapy: The next decade. *Behavior Therapy, 11*, 315-328.

Barnett, L. R., & Nietzel, M. T. (1979). Relationship of instrumental and affectional behaviors and self-esteem to marital satisfaction in distressed and nondistressed couples. *Journal of Consulting and Clinical Psychology, 47*, 946-957.

Barnett, P. A., & Gotlib, I. H. (1988). Psychosocial functioning and depression: Distinguishing among antecedents, concomitants, and consequences. *Psychological Bulletin, 104*, 97-126.

Barthe, D. G., & Hammen, C. L. (1981). The attributional model of depression: A naturalistic extension. *Personality and Social Psychology Bulletin, 7*, 53-58.

Baucom, D. H., & Epstein, N. (1990). *Cognitive-behavioral marital therapy.* New York: Brunner/Mazel.

Beach, S. R. H., Abramson, L. Y., & Levine, F. M. (1981). Attributional reformulation of learned helplessness and depression: Therapeutic implications. In J. F. Clarkin & H. I. Glazer (Eds.), *Depression: Behavioral and directive intervention strategies.* New York: Garland.

Beach, S. R. H., Arias, I., & O'Leary, K. D. (1987). The relationship of marital satisfaction and social support to depressive symptomatology. *Journal of Psychopathology and Behavioral Assessment, 8*, 305-316.

Beach, S. R. H., Arias, I., & O'Leary, K. D. (1988, August). *Life events, marital discord, and depressive symptomatology: Longitudinal relationships.* Paper presented at the 96th annual meeting of the American Psychological Association, Atlanta.

Beach, S. R. H., Arias, I., & O'Leary, K. D. (1989). *Marriage and depression: Longitudinal relationships.* Unpublished manuscript, University of Georgia.

Beach, S. R. H., & Bauserman, S. A. K. (1990). Enhancing the effectiveness of marital therapy. In F. D. Fincham & T. N. Bradbury (Eds.), *The psychology of marriage.* New York: Guilford.

Beach, S. R. H., & Broderick, J. E. (1983). Commitment: A variable in women's response to marital therapy. *American Journal of Family Therapy, 11*, 16-24.

Beach, S. R. H., Jouriles, E. N., & O'Leary, K. D. (1985). Extramarital sex: Impact on depression and commitment in couples seeking marital therapy. *Journal of Sex and Marital Therapy, 11*, 99-108.

Beach, S. R. H., & Nelson, G. M. (1989, August). *Marital discord and depression: Is depression associated with a distinct type of marital discord?* Paper presented at the 97th annual meeting of the American Psychological Association, New Orleans.

Beach, S. R. H., & Nelson, G. M. (1990). Pursuing research on major psychopathology from a contextual perspective: The example of depression and marital discord. In G. Brody & I. E. Sigel (Eds.), *Family research* (Vol. II). Hillsdale, NJ: Erlbaum.

Beach, S. R. H., Nelson, G. M., & O'Leary, K. D. (1988). Cognitive and marital factors in depression. *Journal of Psychopathology and Behavioral Assessment, 10*, 93-105.

Beach, S. R. H., & O'Leary, K. D. (1985). The current status of outcome research in marital therapy. In L. L'Abate (Ed.), *Handbook of family psychology and psychotherapy*. Homewood, IL: Dow Jones-Irwin.

Beach, S. R. H., & O'Leary, K. D. (1986). The treatment of depression occurring in the context of marital discord. *Behavior Therapy, 17*, 43-49.

Beach, S. R. H., & Tesser, A. (1987). Love in marriage: A cognitive account. In R. J. Sternberg & M. J. Barnes (Eds.), *The anatomy of love*. New Haven, CT: Yale University Press.

Beach, S. R. H., Winters, K. C., & Weintraub, S. (1986). Marital dissolution and distress in a psychiatric population: A longitudinal design. *Behavioral Residential Treatment, 1*, 217-229.

Beck, A. T. (1963). Thinking and depression: I. Idiosyncratic content and cognitive distortions. *Archives of General Psychiatry, 9*, 324-333.

Beck, A. T. (1967). *Depression: Clinical, experimental, and theoretical aspects*. Philadelphia: University of Pennsylvania Press.

Beck, A. T. (1972). *Depression: Causes and treatment*. Philadelphia: University of Pennsylvania Press.

Beck, A. T. (1976). *Cognitive therapy and the emotional disorders*. New York: International Universities Press.

Beck, A. T., Brown, G., Steer, R. A., Eidelson, J. I., & Riskind, J. H. (1987). Differentiating anxiety and depression: A test of the cognitive content-specificity hypothesis. *Journal of Abnormal Psychology, 96*, 179-183.

Beck, A. T., & Hurvich, M. S. (1959). Psychological correlates of depression. 1. Frequency of "masochistic" dream content in a private practice sample. *Psychosomatic Medicine, 21*, 50-55.

Beck, A. T., Rush, A. J., Shaw, B. F., & Emery, G. (1979). *Cognitive therapy of depression*. New York: Guilford.

Beck, A. T., Steer, R. A., & Garbin, M. G. (1988). Psychometric properties of the Beck Depression Inventory: Twenty-five years of evaluation. *Clinical Psychology Review, 8*, 77-100.

Beiser, M. (1985). A study of depression among traditional Africans, urban North Americans, and Southeast Asian refugees. In A. Kleinman & B. Good (Eds.), *Culture and depression: Studies in the anthropology and cross-cultural psychiatry of affect and disorder*. Berkeley: University of California Press.

Beiser, M., & Flemming, J. A. E. (1986). Measuring psychiatric disorder among Southeast Asian refugees. *Psychological Medicine, 16*, 627-639.

Bem, D. J. (1972). Self-perception theory. In L. Berkowitz (Ed.), *Advances in experimental social psychology* (Vol. 6). New York: Academic.

Benassi, V.A., Sweeney, P. D., & Dufour, C. L. (1988). Is there a relationship between locus of control orientation and depression? *Journal of Abnormal Psychology, 97*, 357-367.

Berg, R., Franzen, M., & Wedding, D. (1987). *Screening for brain impairment: A manual for mental health practice*. New York: Springer.

Bernard, J. (1972). *The future of marriage*. New York: World.

Biglan, A., Hops, H., & Sherman, L. (1988). Coercive family processes and maternal depression. In R. D. Peters & R. J. McMahon (Eds.), *Social learning and systems approaches to marriage and the family*. New York: Brunner/Mazel.

Biglan, A., Hops, H., Sherman, L., Friedman, L. S., Arthur, J., & Osteen, V. (1985). Problem solving interactions of depressed women and their husbands. *Behavior Therapy, 16*, 431-451.

Biglan, A., Rothlind, J., Hops, H., & Sherman, L. (1989). Impact of distressed and aggressive behavior. *Journal of Abnormal Psychology, 98*, 218-228.

Billings, A. (1979). Conflict resolution in distressed and nondistressed married couples. *Journal of Consulting and Clinical Psychology, 47*, 368–376.

Billings, A. G., & Moos, R. H. (1982). Psychosocial theory and research on depression: An integrative framework and review. *Clinical Psychology Review, 2*, 213–237.

Birchler, G. R., Weiss, R. L., & Vincent, J. P. (1975). Multimethod analysis of social reinforcement exchange between maritally distressed and nondistressed spouse and stranger dyads. *Journal of Personality and Social Psychology, 31*, 349–360.

Blanchard, C. G., Blanchard, E. G., & Becker, J. V. (1976). The young widow: Depressive symptomatology through the grief process. *Psychiatry, 9*, 394–399.

Bloom, B., Asher, S. J., & White, S. W. (1978). Marital disruption as a stressor: A review and analysis. *Psychological Bulletin, 85*, 867–894.

Boswell, P. C., & Murray, E. J. (1981). Depression, schizophrenia, and social attraction. *Journal of Consulting and Clinical Psychology, 49*, 641–647.

Bothwell, S., & Weissman, M. M. (1977). Social impairments four years after an acute depressive episode. *American Journal of Orthopsychiatry, 47*, 231–237.

Boyd, J. H., & Klerman, G. L. (1978). Epidemiology of affective disorders: A reexamination and future directions. *Archives of General Psychiatry, 38*, 1039–1046.

Boyd, J. H., & Weissman, M. M. (1981). Epidemiology of affective disorders: A reexamination and future directions. *Archives of General Psychiatry, 38*, 1039–1046.

Brannon, S. E., & Nelson, R. O. (1987). Contingency management treatment of outpatient unipolar depression: A comparison of reinforcement and extinction. *Journal of Consulting and Clinical Psychology, 55*, 117–119.

Brehm, S. S. (1984). Social support processes. In J. C. Masters & K. Yarkin-Levin (Eds.), *Boundary areas in social and developmental psychology*. Orlando, FL: Academic.

Broderick, J. E., & O'Leary, K. D. (1986). Contributions of affect, attitudes and behavior to marital satisfaction. *Journal of Consulting and Clinical Psychology, 54*, 514–517.

Brown, G. W. (1979). A three factor causal model of depression. In J. E. Barrett, R. Rose, & G. L. Klerman (Eds.), *Stress and mental disorder*. New York: Raven.

Brown, G. W., Andrews, B., Harris, T., Adler, Z., & Bridge, L. (1986). Social support, self-esteem and depression. *Psychological Medicine, 16*, 813–831.

Brown, G. W., & Harris, T. (1978). *Social origins of depression: A study of psychiatric disorders in women*. New York: Free Press.

Brown, G. W., & Harris, T. (1986). Establishing causal links: The Bedford College studies of depression. In H. Katschnig (Ed.), *Life events and psychiatric disorders: Controversial issues*. Cambridge, UK: Cambridge University Press.

Brown, G. W., Harris, T. O., & Bifulco, A. (1986). Long-term effects of early loss of parent. In M. Rutter, C. E. Izard, & P. B. Read (Eds.), *Depression in young people: Developmental and clinical perspectives*. New York: Guilford.

Brown, G. W., & Prudo, R. (1981). Psychiatric disorder in a rural and an urban population: 1. Aetiology of depression. *Psychological Medicine, 11*, 581–599.

Brown, R. A., & Lewinsohn, P. M. (1984). A psychoeducational approach to the treatment of depression: Comparison of group, individual, and minimal contact procedures. *Journal of Consulting and Clinical Psychology, 52*, 774–783.

Bullock, R., Siegel, R., Weissman, M. M., & Paykel, E. S. (1972). The weeping wife: Marital relations of depressed women. *Journal of Marriage and the Family, 34*, 488–495.

Burchill, S. A. L., & Stiles, W. B. (1988). Interactions of depressed college students with their roommates: Not necessarily negative. *Journal of Personality and Social Psychology, 55*, 410–419.

Burgess, R. L. (1981). Relationships in the marriage and family. In S. W. Duck & R. Gilmore (Eds.), *Personal relationships, 1: Studying personal relationships*. New York: Academic.

Burleson, B. R., & Samter, W. (1985). Consistencies in theoretical and naive evaluations of comforting messages. *Communication Monographs, 52*, 103-123.

Burton, R. (1973). *The anatomy of melancholia.* New York: AMS Press. (Original work published 1624, reprinted 1893)

Cameron, O. G. (1987). *Presentations of depression: Depressive symptoms in medical and other psychiatric disorders.* New York: Wiley.

Caplan, G. Support systems. (1974). In G. Caplan (Ed.), *Support systems and community mental health: Lectures on concept development.* New York: Behavioral Publications.

Carroll, B.J., Feinberg, M., Greden, J. F., Tarika, J., Albala, A. A., Haskett, R. F., James, N. M., Kronfol, Z., Lohr, N., Steiner, M., de Vigne, J. P., & Young, E. (1981). A specific laboratory test for the diagnosis of melancholia. *Archives of General Psychiatry, 38*, 15-22.

Carver, C. S., Blaney, P. H., & Scheier, M. F. (1979). Focus of attention, chronic expectancy, and responses to a feared stimulus. *Journal of Personality and Social Psychology, 37*, 1186-1195.

Carver, C. S., & Ganellen, R. J. (1983). Depression and components of self-punitiveness: High standards, self-criticism, and over-generalization. *Journal of Abnormal Psychology, 92*, 330-337.

Chaikin, A. L., Derlega, V. J., & Miller, S. J. (1976). Effects of room environment on self-disclosure in a counseling analogue. *Journal of Counseling Psychology, 23*, 479-481.

Charney, E. A., & Weissman, M. M. (1988). Epidemiology of depressive and manic syndromes. In A. Georgotas & R. Cancro (Eds.), *Depression and mania.* New York: Elsevier.

Chelune, G. J., Sultan, F. E., Vosk, B. N., Ogden, J. K., & Waring, E. M. (1984). Self-disclosure patterns in clinical and nonclinical couples. *Journal of Clinical Psychology, 40*, 213-215.

Christensen, A. (1987). Detection of conflict patterns in couples. In K. Hahlweg & M. J. Goldstein (Eds.), *Understanding major mental disorder: The contribution of family interaction research.* New York: Family Press.

Clarkin, J. F., Haas, G. L., & Glick, I. D. (1988). Inpatient family intervention. In J. F. Clarkin, G. L. Haas, & I. D. Glick (Eds.), *Affective disorders and the family: Assessment and treatment.* New York: Guilford.

Clayton, P. J. (1982). Bereavement. In E. S. Paykel (Ed.), *Handbook of affective disorders.* New York: Guilford.

Clayton, P. J., Halikas, J. A., & Maurice, W. L. (1982). The depression of widowhood. *British Journal of Psychiatry, 120*, 71-78.

Cochran, S. D., & Peplau, L. A. (1985). Value orientations in heterosexual relationships. *Psychology of Women Quarterly, 9*, 477-488.

Cochrane, R. (1988). Marriage, separation, and divorce. In S. Fisher & J. Reason (Eds.), *Handbook of life stress, cognition and health.* New York: Wiley.

Coleman, R. E., & Miller, A. G. (1975). The relationship between depression and marital maladjustment in a clinic population: A multitrait-multimethod study. *Journal of Consulting and Clinical Psychology, 43*, 647-651.

Cook, M. L., & Peterson, C. (1986). Depressive irrationality. *Cognitive Therapy and Research, 10*, 293-298.

Costello, C. G. (1982). Social factors associated with depression: A retrospective community study. *Psychological Medicine, 12*, 329-339.

Coyne, J. C. (1976). Toward an interactional description of depression. *Psychiatry, 39*, 28-40.

Coyne, J. C. (1988). Strategic therapy. In J. F. Clarkin, G. L. Haas, & I. D. Glick (Eds.), *Affective disorders and the family: Assessment and treatment.* New York: Guilford.

Coyne, J. C. (1989). Employing therapeutic paradox in the treatment of depression. In L. M. Ascher (Ed.), *Therapeutic paradox.* New York: Guilford.

Coyne, J. C., Kessler, R. C., Tal, M., Turnbull, J., Wortman, C. B., & Greeden, J. F. (1987). Living with a depressed person. *Journal of Consulting and Clinical Psychology, 55*, 347–352.

Craighead, W. E., Kennedy, R. E., Raczynski, J. M., & Dow, M. G. (1984). Affective disorders—Unipolar. In S. M. Turner & M. Hersen (Eds.), *Adult psychopathology: A behavioral perspective.* New York: Wiley.

Cutrona, C. E. (1984). Social support and stress in the transition to parenthood. *Journal of Abnormal Psychology, 43*, 378–390.

Davis, J. M., Koslow, S. H., Gibbons, R. D., Maas, J. W., Bowden, C. L., Casper, R., Hanin, I., Javaid, J. I., Chang, S. S., & Stokes, P. E. (1988). Cerebrospinal fluid and urinary biogenic amines in depressed patients and healthy controls. *Archives of General Psychiatry, 45*, 705–717.

DeMonbreun, B. G., & Craighead, W. E. (1977). Distortion of perception and recall of positive and neutral feedback in depression. *Cognitive Therapy and Research, 1*, 311–329.

Denoff, M. S. (1982). The differentiation of supportive functions among network members: An empirical inquiry. *Journal of Social Service Research, 5*, 45–59.

Dent, J., & Teasdale, J. D. (1988). Negative cognition and the persistence of depression. *Journal of Abnormal Psychology, 97*, 29–34.

Diener, E. (1984). Subjective well-being. *Psychological Bulletin, 95*, 542–575.

DiMascio, A., Weissman, M. M., Prusoff, B. A., Neu, C., Zwilling, M., & Klerman, G. L. (1979). Differential symptom reduction by drugs and psychotherapy in acute depression. *Archives of General Psychiatry, 36*, 1450–1456.

Dobson, K. S. (1989). A meta-analysis of the efficacy of cognitive therapy for depression. *Journal of Consulting and Clinical Psychology, 57*, 414–419.

Dobson, K. S., Jacobson, N. S., & Victor, J. (1988). Integration of cognitive therapy and behavioral marital therapy. In J. F. Clarkin, G. L. Haas, & I. D. Glick (Eds.), *Affective disorders and the family: Assessment and treatment.* New York: Guilford.

Duval, S., & Wicklund, R. A. (1972). *A theory of objective self-awareness.* New York: Academic.

D'Zurilla, T. J. (1986). *Problem-solving therapy: A social competence approach to clinical intervention.* New York: Springer.

D'Zurilla, T. J., & Goldfried, M. R. (1971). Problem solving and behavior modification. *Journal of Abnormal Psychology, 78*, 107–126.

Egan, G. (1986). *The skilled helper: A systematic approach to effective helping.* Monterey, CA: Brooks-Cole.

Eidelson, R. J., & Epstein, N. (1982). Cognition and relationship maladjustment: Development of a measure of dysfunctional relationship beliefs. *Journal of Consulting and Clinical Psychology, 50*, 715–720.

Elkin, I., Shea, M. T., Watkins, J. T., Imber, S. D., Sotsky, S. M., Collins, J. F., Glass, D. R., Pilkonis, P. A., Leber, W. R., Docherty, J. P., Fiester, S. J., & Parloff, M. B. (1989). National Institute of Mental Health Treatment of Depression Collaborative Research Program: General effectiveness of treatments. *Archives of General Psychiatry, 46*, 971–982.

Ellgring, H., Wagner, H., & Clarke, A. H. (1980). Psychopathological states and their effects on speech and gaze behaviour. In H. Giles, W. P. Robinson, & P. M. Smith (Eds.), *Language: Social psychological perspectives.* Oxford, UK: Pergamon.

Endicott, J., & Spitzer, R. L. (1978). A diagnostic interview: The Schedule for Affective Disorders and Schizophrenia. *Archives of General Psychiatry, 35,* 837-844.

Epstein, N. (1985). Depression and marital dysfunction: Cognitive and behavioral linkages. *International Journal of Mental Health, 13,* 86-104.

Epstein, N., Schlesinger, S. E., & Dryden, W. (Eds.). (1988). *Cognitive-behavioral therapy with families.* New York: Brunner/Mazel.

Epstein, S. (1982). Conflict and stress. In L. Goldberger & S. Breznitz (Eds.), *Handbook of stress: Theoretical and clinical aspects.* New York: Free Press.

Falloon, I. R. H., Hole, V., Mulroy, L., Norris, L. J., & Pembleton, T. (1988). Behavioral family therapy. In J. F. Clarkin, G. L. Haas, & I. D. Glick (Eds.), *Affective disorders and the family: Assessment and treatment.* New York: Guilford.

Filsinger, E. E., & Thoma, S. J. (1988). Behavioral antecedents of relationship stability and adjustment: A five-year longitudinal study. *Journal of Marriage and the Family, 50,* 785-795.

Fincham, F. (1985). Attributions in close relationships. In J. H. Harvey & G. Weary (Eds.), *Attribution: Basic issues and applications.* New York: Academic.

Fincham, F., Beach, S. R. H., & Nelson, G. (1987). Attribution process in distressed and nondistressed couples: 3. Causal and responsibility attributions for spouse behavior. *Cognitive Therapy and Research, 11,* 71-86.

Fincham, F. D., & Bradbury, T. N. (1987a). The assessment of marital quality: A reevaluation. *Journal of Marriage and the Family, 49,* 797-809.

Fincham, F. D., & Bradbury, T. N. (1987b). Cognitive processes and conflict in close relationships: An attribution efficacy model. *Journal of Personality and Social Psychology, 53,* 1106-1118.

Fincham, F. D., Bradbury, T. N., & Grych, J. H. (1990). Conflict in close relationships: The role of intrapersonal phenomena. In S. Graham & V. Folks (Eds.), *Attribution theory: Applications to achievement, mental health, and interpersonal conflict.* Hillsdale: NJ: Erlbaum.

Fischer, S., & Reason, J. T. (1988). *Handbook of life stress, cognition, and health.* New York: Wiley.

Fitzpatrick, M. A. (1987). Marriage and verbal intimacy. In V. J. Derlega & J. Berg (Eds.), *Self-disclosure: Theory, research, and therapy.* New York: Plenum.

Floyd, F., & Markman, H. (1983). Observational biases in spouse observation: Toward a cognitive/behavioral model of marriage. *Journal of Consulting and Clinical Psychology, 51,* 450-457.

Foley, S. H., Rounsaville, B. J., Weissman, M. M., Sholomskas, D., & Chevron, E. (in press). Individual versus conjoint interpersonal psychotherapy for depressed patients with marital disputes. *International Journal of Family Psychiatry.*

Folkman, S., & Lazarus, R. S. (1986). Stress processes and depressive symptomatology. *Journal of Abnormal Psychology, 95,* 107-113.

Folkman, S., & Lazarus, R. S. (1988). Coping as a mediator of emotion. *Journal of Personality and Social Psychology, 54,* 466-475.

Freud, S. (1986). Mourning and melancholia. In J. Coyne (Ed.), *Essential papers on depression.* New York: New York University Press. (Original work published 1917)

Friedman, A. (1975). Interaction of drug therapy with marital therapy in depressive patients. *Archives of General Psychiatry, 32,* 619-637.

Gelman, D. (1987, May 4). Depression. *Newsweek,* 48-52; 54-57.

Gershon, E. S., Hamovit, J., Guroff, J. J., Dibble, E., Leckman, J. F., Sceery, W., Targum, S. D., Nurnberger, J. I., Jr., Goldin, L. R., Bunney, W. E., Jr. (1982). A family study of schizoaffective, bipolar I, biopolar II, unipolar, and normal control probands. *Archives of General Psychiatry, 39,* 1157-1167.

Glass, D. C., & Singer, J. E. (1972). *Urban stress: Experiments on noise and social stressors.* New York: Academic.

Glick, P. G. (1984). How American families are changing. *American Demographics, 6,* 20–27.

Goetz, R. R., Puig-Antich, J., Ryan, N., Rabinovich, H., Ambrosini, P. J., Nelson, B., & Krawiec, V. (1987). Electroencephalographic sleep of adolescents with major depression and normal controls. *Archives of General Psychiatry, 44,* 61–68.

Gold, M. S. (1987). *The good news about depression: Cures and treatments in the new age of psychiatry.* New York: Villard.

Goldberger, L., & Breznitz, S. (Eds.). (1982). *Handbook of stress: Theoretical and clinical aspects.* New York: Free Press.

Goldstein, M. J. (1985). Family factors that antedate the onset of schizophrenia and related disorders: The results of a fifteen year prospective longitudinal study. *Acta Psychiatrica Scandinavica, 71,* 7–18.

Gotlib, I. H., & Asarnow, R. F. (1979). Interpersonal and impersonal problem-solving skills in mildly and clinically depressed university students. *Journal of Consulting and Clinical Psychology, 47,* 86–95.

Gotlib, I. H., & Colby, C. A. (1987). *Treatment of depression: An interpersonal systems approach.* New York: Pergamon.

Gotlib, I. H., & Whiffen, V. E. (1989). Depression and marital functioning: An examination of specificity and gender differences. *Journal of Abnormal Psychology, 98,* 23–30.

Gottman, J. M. (1979). *Marital interaction: Experimental investigations.* New York: Academic.

Gottman, J. M. (1980). Consistency of nonverbal affect and affect reciprocity in marital interaction. *Journal of Consulting and Clinical Psychology, 48,* 711–717.

Gottman, J. M., & Krokoff, L. J. (1989). Marital interaction and satisfaction: A longitudinal view. *Journal of Consulting and Clinical Psychology, 57,* 47–52.

Gottman, J. M., Markman, H., & Notarius, C. (1977). The topography of marital conflict: A sequential analysis of verbal and nonverbal behavior. *Journal of Marriage and the Family, 39,* 461–477.

Gottman, J. M., Notarius, C., Gonso, J., & Markman, H. (1976). *A couple's guide to communication.* Champaign, IL: Research Press.

Gove, W. R., Hughes, M., & Style, C. B. (1983). Does marriage have positive effects on the psychological well-being of the individual? *Journal of Health and Social Behavior, 24,* 122–131.

Greden, J. F., & Carroll, B. J. (1980). Decrease in speech pause times with treatment of endogenous depression. *Biological Psychiatry, 15,* 575–587.

Green, R. A., & Murray, E. J. (1973). Instigation to aggression as a function of self-disclosure and threat to self-esteem. *Journal of Consulting and Clinical Psychology, 40,* 440–443.

Gurin, G., Veroff, J., & Feld, S. (1960). *Americans view their health: A nationwide interview study.* New York: Basic Books.

Gurtman, M. B. (1986). Depression and the response of others: Reevaluating the reevaluation. *Journal of Abnormal Psychology, 95,* 99–101.

Guthrie, D. M. (1988). *Husbands' and wives' expressiveness: An analysis of self-evaluations, perceptions of expressiveness and emotional cues.* Unpublished doctoral dissertation, University of Queensland, St. Lucia, Australia.

Hafner, R. J. (1986). *Marriage and mental illness: A sex-roles perspective.* New York: Guilford.

Hafner, R. J., Badenoch, A., Fisher, J., & Swift, H. (1983). Spouse-aided versus individual therapy in persisting psychiatric disorders: A systematic comparison. *Family Process, 22,* 385–399.

Hagnell, O., Lanke, J., Rorsman, B., & Ojesjo, L. (1982). Are we entering an age of melancholy? Depressive illness in a prospective epidemiological study over 25 years: The Lundby study, Sweden. *Psychological Medicine, 12*, 279–289.

Hahlweg, K., & Markman, H. J. (1988). The effectiveness of behavioral marital therapy: Empirical status of behavioral techniques in preventing and alleviating marital distress. *Journal of Consulting and Clinical Psychology, 56*, 440–447.

Hales, R. E. (1986). The diagnosis and treatment of psychiatric disorders in medically ill patients. *Military Medicine, 151*(11), 587–595.

Hamilton, M. (1982). Symptoms and assessment of depression. In E. S. Paykel (Ed.), *Handbook of affective disorders.* New York: Guilford.

Hammen, C. L. (1985). Predicting depression: A cognitive-behavioral perspective. In P. C. Kendall (Ed.), *Advances in cognitive-behavioral research and therapy* (Vol. 4). Orlando, FL: Academic.

Hammen, C. L., Ellicott, A., Gitlin, M., & Jamison, K. R. (1989). Sociotropy/autonomy and vulnerability to specific life events in patients with unipolar and bipolar disorders. *Journal of Abnormal Psychology, 98*, 154–160.

Hautzinger, M., Linden, M., & Hoffman, N. (1982). Distressed couples with and without a depressed partner: An analysis of their verbal interaction. *Journal of Behavior Therapy and Experimental Psychiatry, 13*, 307–314.

Hawton, K. (1986). *Suicide and attempted suicide among children and adolescents.* Beverly Hills, CA: Sage.

Heider, F. (1958). *The psychology of interpersonal relations.* New York: Wiley.

Heiman, J. R., LoPiccolo, L. J., & LoPiccolo, J. (1976). *Becoming orgasmic: A sexual growth program for women.* Englewood Cliffs, NJ: Prentice-Hall.

Heller, K., Swindle, R. W., Jr., & Dusenbury, L. (1986). Component social support processes: Comments and integration. *Journal of Consulting and Clinical Psychology, 54*, 466–470.

Hendrick, S. S. (1981). Self-disclosure and marital satisfaction. *Journal of Personality and Social Psychology, 40*, 1150–1159.

Hinchliffe, M. K., Hooper, D., & Roberts, J. (1978). *The melancholy marriage: Depression in marriage and psychosocial approaches to therapy.* New York: Wiley.

Hinchliffe, M., Lancashire, M. H., & Roberts, F. J. (1970). Eye contact and depression: A preliminary report. *British Journal of Psychiatry, 117*, 571–572.

Hirschfeld, R. M. A., & Cross, C. K. (1982). Epidemiology of affective disorders. *Archives of General Psychiatry, 39*, 35–46.

Hoberman, H. M., & Lewinsohn, P. M. (1985). The behavioral treatment of depression. In E. E. Beckham & W. R. Leber (Eds.), *Handbook of depression: Treatment, assessment, and research.* Homewood, IL: Dorsey.

Hobfall, S. E. (Ed.). (1986). *Stress, social support, and women.* Washington, DC: Hemisphere.

Hollon, S. D., & Beck, A. T. (1978). Psychotherapy and drug therapy: Comparisons and combinations. In S. L. Garfield & A. E. Bergin (Eds.), *Handbook of psychotherapy and behavior change: An empirical analysis* (2nd ed.). New York: Wiley.

Hollon, S. D., & Beck, A. T. (1979). Cognitive therapy of depression. In P. C. Kendall & S. D. Hollon (Eds.), *Cognitive-behavioral interventions: Theory, research, and procedures.* New York: Academic.

Hollon, S. D., & Kendall, P. C. (1980). Cognitive self-statements in depression: Development of an Automatic Thoughts Questionnaire. *Cognitive Therapy and Research, 4*, 383–395.

Holmes, T. H., & Rahe, R. H. (1967). The social readjustment rating scale. *Journal of Psychosomatic Research, 11*, 213–218.

Hooley, J. M. (1986). Expressed emotion and depression: Interactions between patients and high- vs. low-expressed-emotion spouses. *Journal of Abnormal Psychology, 95,* 237–246.

Hooley, J. M., & Hahlweg, K. (1985). The marriages and interaction patterns of depressed patients and their spouses: Comparing high and low EE dyads. In M. J. Goldstein, I. Hand, & K. Hahlweg (Eds.), *Treatment of schizophrenia: Family assessment and intervention.* Heidelberg and Berlin: Springer-Verlag.

Hooley, J. M., Orley, J., & Teasdale, J. D. (1986). Levels of expressed emotion and relapse in depressed patients. *British Journal of Psychiatry, 148,* 642–647.

Hooley, J. M., Richters, J. E., Weintraub, S., & Neale, J. M. (1987). Psychopathology and marital distress: The positive side of positive symptoms. *Journal of Abnormal Psychology, 96,* 27–33.

Hooley, J. M., & Teasdale, J. D. (1989). Predictors of relapse in unipolar depressives: Expressed emotion, marital distress, and perceived criticism. *Journal of Abnormal Psychology, 98,* 229–235.

Hops, H., Biglan, A., Sherman, L., Arthur, J., Friedman, L., & Osteen, V. (1987). Home observation of family interactions of depressed women. *Journal of Consulting and Clinical Psychology, 55,* 341–346.

House, J. S., Landis, K. R., & Umberson, D. (1988). Social relationships and health. *Science, 241,* 540–545.

Ilfeld, F. W., Jr. (1976). Methodological issues in relating psychiatric symptoms to social stressors. *Psychological Reports, 39,* 1251–1258.

Ilfeld, F. W., Jr. (1977). Current social stressors and symptoms of depression. *American Journal of Psychiatry, 134,* 161–166.

Ingram, R. E., Lumrey, A. E., Cruet, D., & Sieber, W. (1987). Attentional processes in depressive disorders. *Cognitive Therapy and Research, 11,* 351–360.

Jacobson, N. S. (1985, August). *Combining marital therapy with individual therapy in the treatment of depression.* Paper presented at the 93rd annual meeting of the American Psychological Association, Los Angeles.

Jacobson, N. S. (1989). The maintenance of treatment gains following social learning–based marital therapy. *Behavior Therapy, 20,* 325–336.

Jacobson, N. S., Follette, W. C., & McDonald, D. W. (1982). Reactivity to positive and negative behavior in distressed and nondistressed married couples. *Journal of Consulting and Clinical Psychology, 50,* 706–714.

Jacobson, N. S., Follette, W. C., & Pagel, M. (1986). Predicting who will benefit from behavioral marital therapy. *Journal of Consulting and Clinical Psychology, 54,* 518–522.

Jacobson, N. S., Holtzworth-Munroe, A., & Schmaling, K. B. (1989). Marital therapy and spouse involvement in the treatment of depression, agoraphobia, and alcoholism. *Journal of Consulting and Clinical Psychology, 57,* 5–10.

Jacobson, N. S., & Margolin, G. (1979). *Marital therapy: Strategies based on social learning and behavior exchange principles.* New York: Brunner/Mazel.

Jacobson, N. S., Schmaling, K. B., & Holtzworth-Munroe, A. (1987). Component analysis of behavioral marital therapy: 2-year follow-up and prediction of relapse. *Journal of Marital and Family Therapy, 13,* 187–195.

Jacobson, N. S., Schmaling, K. B., Holtzworth-Munroe, A., Katt, J. L., Wood, L. F., & Follette, V. M. (1989). Research structured versus clinically flexible versions of social learning based marital therapy. *Behaviour Research and Therapy, 27,* 173–180.

Jacobson, N. S., Schmaling, K. B., Salusky, S., Follette, V., & Dobson, K. (1987, November). *Marital therapy as an adjunct treatment for depression.* Paper presented at the 21st annual meeting of the Association for Advancement of Behavior Therapy, Boston.

Jacobson, N. S., Waldron, H., & Moore, D. (1980). Toward a behavioral profile of marital distress. *Journal of Consulting and Clinical Psychology, 48*, 696–703.

Joyce, P. R., & Paykel, E. S. (1989). Predictors of drug response in depression. *Archives of General Psychiatry, 46*, 89–99.

Kahn, J., Coyne, J. C., & Margolin, G. (1985). Depression and marital disagreement: The social construction of despair. *Journal of Social and Personal Relationships, 2*, 447–461.

Kandel, D. B., & Davies, M. (1982). Epidemiology of depressed mood in adolescents. *Archives of General Psychiatry, 39*, 1205–1212.

Kanfer, F. (1970). Self-monitoring: Methodological limitations and clinical applications. *Journal of Consulting and Clinical Psychology, 35*, 148–152.

Kanner, A. D., Coyne, J. C., & Schaefer, C. (1981). Comparison of two modes of stress measurement: Daily hassles and uplifts versus major life events. *Journal of Behavioral Medicine, 4*, 1–39.

Kaplan, H. S. (1974). *The new sex therapy: Active treatment of sexual dysfunctions.* New York: Brunner/Mazel.

Kazak, A. E., Jarmas, A., Snitzer, L. (1988). The assessment of marital satisfaction: An evaluation of the Dyadic Adjustment Scale. *Journal of Family Psychology, 2*, 82–91.

Kendler, K. S., Heath, A. C., Martin, N. G., & Eaves, L. J. (1987). Symptoms of anxiety and symptoms of depression. *Archives of General Psychiatry, 44*, 451–457.

Kessler, R. C., & McLeod, J. (1985). Social support and psychological distress in community surveys. In S. Cohen & S. Syme (Eds.), *Social support and health.* Orlando, FL: Academic.

Kessler, R. C., Price, R. H., & Wortman, C. B. (1985). Social factors in psychopathology: Stress, social support, and coping processes. In M. R. Rosenzweig & L. W. Porter (Eds.), *Annual review of psychology* (Vol. 36). Palo Alto, CA: Annual Reviews.

Klein, M. (1940). Mourning and its relation to manic–depressive states. In *Contributions to psychoanalysis, 1921–1945.* London: Hogarth Press.

Kleinman, A. (1988). *Rethinking psychiatry: From cultural category to personal experience.* New York: Free Press.

Klerman, G. L. (1988). The treatment of depressive conditions. In *Perspectives on depressive disorders: A review of recent research.* Rockville, MD: National Institute of Mental Health.

Klerman, G. L., Weissman, M. M., Rounsaville, B. J., & Chevron, E. S. (1984). *Interpersonal psychotherapy of depression.* New York: Basic Books.

Koren, P., Carlton, K., & Shaw, D. (1980). Marital conflict: Relations among behaviors, outcomes, and distress. *Journal of Consulting and Clinical Psychology, 48*, 460–468.

Kovacs, M., & Beck, A. T. (1978). Maladaptive cognitive structures in depression. *American Journal of Psychiatry, 135*, 525–533.

Kovacs, M., Rush, A. J., Beck, A. T., & Hollon, S. D. (1981). Depressed outpatients treated with cognitive therapy or pharmacotherapy: A one year follow-up. *Archives of General Psychiatry, 38*, 33–39.

Krantz, S. E., & Moos, R. H. (1988). Risk factors at intake predict nonremission among depressed patients. *Journal of Consulting and Clinical Psychology, 56*, 863–869.

Kuiper, N. A. (1978). Depression and causal attributions for success and failure. *Journal of Personality and Social Psychology, 36*, 236–246.

Kuiper, N. A., & Olinger, L. J. (1989). Stress and cognitive vulnerability for depression: A self-worth contingency model. In R. W. J. Neufield (Ed.), *Advances in the investigation of psychological stress.* New York: Wiley.

Lange, A. J., & Jakubowski, P. (1976). *Responsible assertive behavior: Cognitive/behavioral procedures for trainers.* Champaign, IL: Research Press.

Lazarus, R. S. (1966). *Psychological stress and the coping process.* New York: McGraw-Hill.

Lazarus, R. S. (1967). Cognitive and personality factors underlying threat and coping. In M. H. Appley & R. A. Trumbull (Eds.), *Psychological stress: Issues in research.* New York: Appleton-Century Crofts.

Lazarus, R. S., & Folkman, S. (1986). Cognitive theories of stress and the issue of circularity. In M. H. Appley & R. A. Trumbull (Eds.), *Dynamics of stress: Physiological, psychological, and social perspectives.* New York: Plenum.

Lehman, D. R., Ellard, J. H., & Wortman, C. B. (1986). Social support for the bereaved: Recipients' and providers' perspectives on what is helpful. *Journal of Consulting and Clinical Psychology, 54,* 438–446.

Levenson, R. W., & Gottman, J. M. (1983). Marital interaction: Physiological linkage and affective exchange. *Journal of Personality and Social Psychology, 45,* 587–597.

Levine, F., & Sandeen, E. (1985). *Conceptualization in psychotherapy: The models of approach.* Hillsdale, NJ: Erlbaum.

Lewinsohn, P. M. (1974). A behavioral approach to depression. In R. J. Friedman & M. M. Katz (Eds.), *The psychology of depression: Contemporary theory and research.* Washington, DC: Winston.

Lewinsohn, P. M., Antonuccio, D. O., Steinmetz, J. L., & Teri, L. (1984). *The coping with depression course.* Eugene, OR: Castalia Publishing.

Lewinsohn, P. M., & Arconad, M. (1981). Behavioral treatment of depression: A social learning approach. In J. F. Clarkin & H. I. Glazer (Eds.), *Depression: Behavioral and directive intervention strategies.* New York: Garland.

Lewinsohn, P. M., & Atwood, G. E. (1969). Depression: A clinical research approach. *Psychotherapy: Theory, Research, and Practice, 6,* 166–171.

Lewinsohn, P. M., Hoberman, H. M., & Rosenbaum, M. (1988). A prospective study of risk factors for unipolar depression. *Journal of Abnormal Psychology, 97,* 251–264.

Lewinsohn, P. M., Hoberman, H. M., Terri, L., & Hautzinger, M. (1985). An integrative theory of depression. In S. Reiss & R. Bootzin (Eds.), *Theoretical issues in behavior therapy.* Orlando, FL: Academic.

Lewinsohn, P. M., & Shaffer, M. (1971). Use of home observations as an integral part of the treatment of depression: Preliminary report and case studies. *Journal of Consulting and Clinical Psychology, 37,* 87–94.

Liberman, R. P., Wheeler, E.G., deVisser, L., Kuehnel, J., & Kuehnel, T. (1980). *Handbook of marital therapy: A positive approach to helping troubled relationships.* New York: Plenum.

Libet, J. M., & Lewinsohn, P. M. (1973). The concept of social skills with special reference to the behavior of depressed persons. *Journal of Consulting and Clinical Psychology, 40,* 304–312.

Lieberman, M. A. (1982). The effects of social supports on responses to stress. In L. Goldberger & S. Breznitz (Eds.), *Handbook of stress.* New York: Free Press.

Lin, N. (1986). Conceptualizing social support. In N. Lin, A. Dean, & W. M. Ensel (Eds.), *Social support, life events, and depression.* Orlando, FL: Academic.

Lin, N., Dean, A., & Ensel, W. M. (Eds.). (1986). *Social support, life events, and depression.* Orlando, FL: Academic.

Lin, N., & Ensel, W. M. (1984). Depression mobility and its social etiology: The role of life events and social support. *Journal of Health and Social Behavior, 25,* 176–188.

Lin, N., Woelfel, M., & Dumin, M. Y. (1986). Gender of the confidant and depression. In

N. Lin, A. Dean, & W. M. Ensel (Eds.), *Social support, life events, and depression.* Orlando, FL: Academic.

Lin, T. Y. (1969). Mental disorders in Taiwan 15 years later. In W. Caudill & T. Y. Lin (Eds.), *Mental health in Asia and the Pacific.* Honolulu: East West Center Press.

Linden, M., Hautzinger, M., & Hoffman, N. (1983). Discriminant analysis of depressive interactions. *Behavior Modification, 7,* 403–422.

Locke, H. J., & Wallace, K. M. (1959). Short marital adjustment and prediction tests: Their reliability and validity. *Marriage and Family Living, 21,* 231–235.

Loeb, A., Beck, A. T., & Diggory, J. (1971). Differential effects of success and failure on depressed and nondepressed patients. *Journal of Nervous and Mental Disease, 152,* 106–114.

Loosen, P. T. (1985). The TRH-induced TSH response in psychiatric patients: A possible neuroendocrine marker. *Psychoneuroendocrinology, 10,* 237–260.

LoPiccolo, J., & LoPiccolo, L. (1978). *Handbook of sex therapy.* New York: Plenum.

Lubin, G. (1965). Adjective checklist for the measurement of depression. *Archives of General Psychiatry, 12,* 57–62.

Madden, M. E., & Janoff-Bulman, R. (1981). Blame, control, and marital satisfaction: Wives' attributions for conflict in marriage. *Journal of Marriage and the Family, 43,* 663–674.

Mandler, G. (1982). Stress and thought processes. In L. Goldberger & S. Breznitz (Eds.), *Handbook of stress: Theoretical and clinical aspects.* New York: Free Press.

Manne, S. L., & Zautra, A. J. (1989). Spouse criticism and support: Their association with coping and psychological adjustment among women with rheumatoid arthritis. *Journal of Personality and Social Psychology, 56,* 608–617.

Margolin, G. (1981). Behavior exchange in happy and unhappy marriages: A family cycle perspective. *Behavior Therapy, 12,* 329–343.

Margolin, G., Talovic, S., & Weinstein, C. D. (1983). Areas of Change Questionnaire: A practical approach to marital assessment. *Journal of Consulting and Clinical Psychology, 51,* 944–955.

Margolin, G., & Wampold, B. E. (1981). Sequential analysis of conflict and accord in distressed and nondistressed marital partners. *Journal of Consulting and Clinical Psychology, 49,* 554–567.

Markman, H. J., Duncan, W., Storaasli,R., & Howes, P. W. (1987). The prediction and prevention of marital distress: A longitudinal investigation. In K. Hahlweg & M. J. Goldstein (Eds.), *Understanding major mental disorder: The contribution of family interaction research.* New York: Family Process.

Marlatt, G. A., & Gordon, J. R. (Eds.). (1985). *Relapse prevention: Maintenance strategies in the treatment of addictive behaviors.* New York: Guilford.

McAdams, D. P., & Vaillant, G. E. (1982). Intimacy motivation and psychosocial adjustment: A longitudinal study. *Journal of Personality Assessment, 46,* 586–593.

McLean, P. D., Ogston, K., & Grauer, L. (1973). A behavioral approach to the treatment of depression. *Journal of Behavior Therapy and Experimental Psychiatry, 4,* 323–330.

Merikangas, K. R. (1984). Divorce and assortative mating among depressed patients. *American Journal of Psychiatry, 141,* 74–76.

Merikangas, K. R., Ranelli, C.J., & Kupfer, D.J. (1979). Marital interaction in hospitalized depressed patients. *Journal of Nervous and Mental Disease, 167,* 689–695.

Metalsky, G. I., Halberstadt, L. J., & Abramson, L. Y. (1987). Vulnerability to depressive mood reactions: Toward a more powerful test of the diathesis–stress and causal mediation of components of the reformulated theory of depression. *Journal of Personality and Social Psychology, 52,* 386–393.

Miklowitz, D. J., Goldstein, M. J., Nuechterlein, K., H., Snyder, K. S., & Doane, J. A. (1986). Expressed emotion, affective style, lithium compliance, and relapse in recent-onset mania. *Psychopharmacology Bulletin, 22,* 628–632.

Millon, T. (1983). *Millon Clinical Multiaxial Inventory manual* (3rd ed.). Minneapolis, MN: National Computer Systems.

Mitchell, R. E., Cronkite, R. C., & Moos, R. H. (1983). Stress, coping and depression among married couples. *Journal of Abnormal Psychology, 92,* 433–448.

Monroe, S. M., Bromet, E. J., Connell, M. M., & Steiner, S. C. (1986). Social support, life events, and depressive symptoms: A one year prospective study. *Journal of Consulting and Clinical Psychology, 54,* 424–431.

Nelson, G.M., & Beach, S. R. H. (in press). Sequential interaction in depression: Effects of depressive behavior on spousal aggression. *Behavior Therapy.*

Nelson, R. E. (1977). Irrational beliefs in depression. *Journal of Consulting and Clinical Psychology, 45,* 1190–1191.

Nelson, R. E., & Craighead, W. E. (1977). Selective recall of positive and negative feedback, self-control behaviors, and depression. *Journal of Abnormal Psychology, 86,* 379–388.

Nezu, A. M., Nezu, C.M., & Perri, M. G. (1989). *Problem-solving therapy for depression: Theory, research and clinical guidelines.* New York: Wiley.

Nezu, A. M., Nezu, C. M., Saraydarian, L., Kalmar, K., & Ronan, G. F. (1986). Social problem solving as a moderating variable between negative life stress and depressive symptoms. *Cognitive Therapy and Research, 10,* 489–498.

Nezu, A. M., & Perri, M. G. (1989). Social problem-solving for unipolar depression: An initial dismantling investigation. *Journal of Consulting and Clinical Psychology, 57,* 408–413.

Nezu, A. M., & Ronan, G. F. (1987). Social problem solving and depression: Deficits in generating alternatives and decision making. *The Southern Psychologist, 3,* 29–34.

Nisbett, R. E., & Ross, L. (1980). *Human inference: Strategies and shortcomings of social judgement.* Englewood Cliffs, NJ: Prentice-Hall.

Nolen-Hoeksema, S. (1987). Sex differences in unipolar depression: Evidence and theory. *Psychological Bulletin, 101,* 259–282.

Noller, P. (1987). Nonverbal communication in marriage. In D. Perlman & S. Duck (Eds.), *Intimate relationships: Development, dynamics, and deterioration.* Beverly Hills, CA: Sage.

Noller, P., & Venardos, C. (1986). Communication awareness in married couples. *Journal of Social and Personal Relationships, 3,* 31–42.

Notarius, C.I., Benson, P. R., Sloane, D., Vanzetti, N. A., & Hornyak, L. M. (1989). Exploring the interface between perception and behavior: An analysis of marital interaction in distressed and nondistressed couples. *Behavioral Assessment, 11,* 39–64.

Novaco, R. W. (1979). The cognitive regulation of anger and stress. In P. C. Kendall & S. D. Hollon (Eds.), *Cognitive-behavioral interventions: Theory, research, and procedures.* Orlando, FL: Academic.

Nurnberger, J. I., & Gershon, E. S. (1982). Genetics. In E. S. Paykel (Ed.), *Handbook of affective disorders.* New York: Guilford.

Oatley, K., & Bolton, W. (1985). A social-cognitive theory of depression in reaction to life events. *Psychological Review, 92,* 372–388.

O'Hara, M. W., & Rehm, L. P. (1979). Self-monitoring, activity levels, and mood in the development and maintenance of depression. *Journal of Abnormal Psychology, 88,* 450–453.

O'Hara, M. W., Rehm, L. P., & Campbell, S. B. (1982). Predicting depressive symptomatology: Cognitive-behavioral models and post-partum depression. *Journal of Abnormal Psychology, 91*, 457–461.

O'Leary, K. D. (1987). *Assessment of marital discord: An integration for research and clinical practice*. Hillsdale, NJ: Erlbaum.

O'Leary, K. D., & Arias, I. (1983). The influence of marital therapy on sexual satisfaction. *Journal of Sex and Marital Therapy, 9*, 171–181.

O'Leary, K. D., Barling, J., Arias, I., Rosenbaum, A., Malone, J., & Tyree, A. (1989). Prevalence and stability of physical aggression between spouses: A longitudinal analysis. *Journal of Consulting and Clinical Psychology, 57*, 263–268.

O'Leary, K. D., & Beach, S. R. H. (1990). Marital therapy: A viable treatment for depression and marital discord. *American Journal of Psychiatry, 147*, 183–186.

O'Leary, K. D., Fincham, F., & Turkewitz, H. (1983). Assessment of positive feelings toward spouse. *Journal of Consulting and Clinical Psychology, 51*, 937–939.

O'Leary, K. D., Sandeen, E., & Beach, S. R. H. (1987, November). *Treatment of suicidal, maritally discordant clients by marital therapy or cognitive therapy*. Paper presented at the 21st annual meeting of the Association for Advancement of Behavior Therapy, Boston.

O'Leary, K. D., & Wilson, G. T. (1987). *Behavior therapy: Application and outcome* (2nd ed.). Englewood Cliffs, NJ: Prentice-Hall.

Olinger, L. J., Kuiper, N. A., & Shaw, B. F. (1987). Dysfunctional attitudes and stressful life events: An interactive model of depression. *Cognitive Therapy and Research, 11*, 25–40.

Orley, J., & Wing, J. K. (1979). Psychiatric disorders in two African villages. *Archives of General Psychiatry, 36*, 513–520.

Parelman, A. (1982). *Emotional intimacy in marriage: A sex-roles perspective*. Ann Arbor: University of Michigan Research Press.

Parker, G., Brown, L., & Blignault, I. (1986). Coping behaviors as predictors of the course of clinical depression. *Archives of General Psychiatry, 43*, 561–565.

Patterson, G. R., & Reid, J. B. (1970). Reciprocity and coercion: Two facets of social systems. In C. Neuringer & J. L. Michael (Eds.), *Behavior modification in clinical psychology*. New York: Appleton-Century-Crofts.

Paykel, E. S. (1979). Recent life events in the development of the depressive disorders. In R. A. Depue (Ed.), *The psychobiology of depressive disorders: Implications for the effects of stress*. New York: Academic.

Paykel, E. S., Myers, J. K., Dienelt, M. N., Klerman, G. L., Lindenthal, J. J., & Pepper, M. P. (1969). Life events and depression: A controlled study. *Archives of General Psychiatry, 21*, 753–760.

Paykel, E. S., Prusoff, B. A., & Myers, J. K. (1975). Suicide attempts and recent life events: A control led comparison. *Archives of General Psychiatry, 32*, 327–333.

Paykel, E. S., & Tanner, J. (1976). Life events, depressive relapse, and maintenance treatment. *Psychological Medicine, 6*, 481–485.

Pearlin, L. I., & Lieberman, M. A. (1979). Social sources of emotional distress. In R. Simmons (Ed.), *Research in community and mental health*. Greenwich, CT: JAI Press.

Pearlin, L.I., Lieberman, M. A., Menaghan, E. G., & Mullan, J. T. (1981). The stress process. *Journal of Health and Social Behavior, 22*, 337–356.

Pearlin, L. I., & Schooler, C. (1978). The structure of coping. *Journal of Health and Social Behavior, 19*, 2–21.

Peck, M. L. (1989). Crisis intervention treatment with chronically and acutely suicidal adolescents. In M. L. Peck, N. L. Farberow, & R. E. Litman (Eds.), *Youth suicide*. New York: Springer.

Pennebaker, J. W. (1988). Confiding traumatic experiences and health. In S. Fisher & J. Reason (Eds.), *Handbook of life stress, cognition, and health*. New York: Wiley.

Perris, C. (1966). A study of bipolar (manic–depressive) and unipolar recurrent depressive psychoses. *Acta Psychiatrica Scandinavica* (Suppl.), *194*, 15–44.

Pyszczynski, T., & Greenberg, J. (1987). Self-regulatory perseveration and the depressive self-focusing style: A self-awareness theory of reactive depression. *Psychological Bulletin, 102*, 122–138.

Rehm, L. P. (1977). A self-control model of depression. *Behavior Therapy, 8*, 787–804.

Rehm, L. P. (1987). Approaches to the prevention of depression in children. In R. F. Munoz (Ed.), *Depression prevention*. Washington, DC: Hemisphere.

Rehm, L. P., & Plakosh, P. (1975). Preference for immediate reinforcement in depression. *Behaviour Research and Experimental Psychiatry, 6*, 101–103.

Renne, K. S. (1970). Correlates of dissatisfaction in marriage. *Journal of Marriage and the Family, 32*, 54–67.

Revenstorf, D., Hahlweg, K., Schindler, L., & Vogel, B. (1984). Interaction analysis of marital conflict. In K. Hahlweg & N. S. Jacobson (Eds.), *Marital interaction: Analysis and modification*. New York: Guilford.

Rice, J., Reich, T., Andreasen, N. C., Endicott, J., Van Eerdewegh, M., Fishman, R., Hirschfeld, R. M. A., & Klerman, G. L. (1987). The familial transmission of bipolar illness. *Archives of General Psychiatry, 44*, 441–447.

Riskind, J. H., Beck, A. T., Berchick, R. J., Brown, G., & Steer, R. A. (1987). Reliability of DSM-III diagnoses for major depression and generalized anxiety disorder using the structured clinical interview for DSM-III. *Archives of General Psychiatry, 44*, 817–820.

Robins, C.J. (1988). Attributions and depression: Why is the literature so inconsistent? *Journal of Personality and Social Psychology, 54*, 880–889.

Robins, C. J., & Block, P. (1988). Personal vulnerability, life events, and depressive symptoms: A test of a specific interactional model. *Journal of Personality and Social Psychology, 54*, 847–852.

Robins, L. N., Helzer, J. E., Weissman, M. M., Orvaschel, H., Gruenberg, E., Burke, J. D., Jr., & Regier, D. A. (1984). Lifetime prevalence of specific psychiatric disorders in three communities. *Archives of General Psychiatry, 41*, 949–958.

Rook, K. S. (1987). Social support vs. companionship: Effects on life stress, loneliness, and evaluations by others. *Journal of Personality and Social Psychology, 52*, 1132–1147.

Rosenblatt, A., & Greenberg, J. (1988). Depression and interpersonal attraction: The role of perceived similarity. *Journal of Personality and Social Psychology, 55*, 112–119.

Ross, L. (1977). The intuitive psychologist and his shortcomings: Distortions in the attribution process. In L. Berkowitz (Ed.), *Advances in experimental social psychology* (Vol. 10). New York: Academic.

Rounsaville, B. J., Weissman, M. M., Prusoff, B. A., & Herceg-Baron, R. L. (1979a). Marital disputes and treatment outcome in depressed women. *Comprehensive Psychiatry, 20*, 483–490.

Rounsaville, B. J., Weissman, M. M., Prusoff, B. A., & Herceg-Baron, R. L. (1979b). Process of psychotherapy among depressed women with marital disputes. *American Journal of Orthopsychiatry, 49*, 505–510.

Roy, A. (1978). Vulnerability factors and depression in women. *British Journal of Psychiatry, 133*, 106–110.

Roy, A., Pickar, D., DeJong, J.., Karoum, F., & Linnoila, M. (1988). Norepinephrine and its metabolites in cerebrospinal fluid, plasma, and urine. *Archives of General Psychiatry, 45*, 849–857.

Ruehlman, L. S., & Wolchik, S. A. (1988). Personal goals and interpersonal support and hindrance as factors in psychological distress and well-being. *Journal of Personality and Social Psychology, 55,* 293–301.

Rush, A. J., Shaw, B., & Khatami, M. (1980). Cognitive therapy of depression: Utilizing the couples system. *Cognitive Therapy and Research, 4,* 103–113.

Rutter, M., Graham, P., Chadwick, O., & Yule, W. (1976). Adolescent turmoil: Fact or fiction? *Journal of Child Psychology and Psychiatry, 17,* 5–56.

Sachar, E. J. (1982). Endocrine abnormalities in depression. In E. S. Paykel (Ed.), *Handbook of affective disorders.* New York: Guilford.

Sager, C.J., Gundlach, R., Kremer, M., Lenz, R., & Royce, J. R. (1968). The married in treatment: Effects of psychoanalysis on the marital state. *Archives of General Psychiatry, 19,* 205–217.

Sandeen, E., O'Leary, K. D., & Beach, S. R. H. (1987, November). *The role of compliance in cognitive therapy or marital therapy for depression.* Paper presented at the 21st annual meeting of the Association for Advancement of Behavior Therapy, Boston.

Sarason, B. R., Shearin, E. N., Pierce, G. R., & Sarason, I. G. (1987). Interrelations of social support measures: Theoretical and practical implications. *Journal of Personality and Social Psychology, 52,* 813–832.

Schaefer, E. S., & Burnett, C. K. (1987). Stability and predictability of quality of women's marital relationships and demoralization. *Journal of Personality and Social Psychology, 53,* 1129–1136.

Scheier, M. F., & Carver, C. S. (1977). Self-focused attention and the experience of emotion: Attraction, repulsion, elation, and depression. *Journal of Personality and Social Psychology, 35,* 625–636.

Schless, A. P., Schwartz, L., Goetz, C., & Mendels, J. (1974). How depressives view the significance of life events. *British Journal of Psychiatry, 125,* 406–410.

Schlesser, M. A. (1986). Neuroendocrine abnormalities in affective disorders. In A. J. Rush & K. Z. Altshuler (Eds.), *Depression: Basic mechanisms, diagnosis, and treatment.* New York: Guilford.

Schneidman, E. S., Farberow, N. L., & Litman, R. E. (1970). *The psychology of suicide.* New York: Science House.

Seligman, M. E. P. (1975). *Helplessness: On depression, development, and death.* San Francisco: Freeman.

Seligman, M. E. P., Abramson, L. Y., Semmel, A., & von Baeyer, C. (1979). Depressive attributional style. *Journal of Abnormal Psychology, 88,* 242–247.

Sharpley, C. F., & Cross, D. G. (1982). A psychometric evaluation of the Spanier Dyadic Adjustment Scale. *Journal of Marriage and the Family, 44,* 739–741.

Shoham-Saloman, V., & Rosenthal, R. (1987). Paradoxical interventions: A meta-analysis. *Journal of Consulting and Clinical Psychology, 55,* 22–28.

Siegman, A. W. (1987). The pacing of speech in depression. In J. D. Maser (Ed.), *Depression and expressive behavior.* Hillsdale, NJ: Erlbaum.

Simons, A. D., Murphy, G. E., Levine, J. L., & Wetzel, R. D. (1986). Cognitive therapy and pharmacotherapy for depression: Sustained improvement over one year. *Archives of General Psychiatry, 43,* 43–48.

Slater, J., & Depue, R. A. (1981). The contribution of environmental events and social support to serious suicide attempts in primary depressive disorder. *Journal of Abnormal Psychology, 90,* 275–285.

Solomon, Z., & Bromet, E. (1982). The role of social factors in affective disorders: An assessment of the vulnerability model of Brown and his colleagues. *Psychological Medicine, 12,* 123–130.

Spanier, G. B. (1976). Measuring dyadic adjustment: New scales for assessing the quality of marriage and similar dyads. *Journal of Marriage and the Family, 38*, 15-28.

Spitzer, R. L., Williams, J. B. W., & Gibbon, M. (1987). *Structured clinical interview for DSM-III-R Personality Disorders (SCID-II, 3-1-87)*. (Available from Biometrics Research Department, New York State Psychiatric Institute, 772 West 168th Street, New York, NY 10032)

Stephens, R. S., Hokanson, J. E., & Welker, R. (1987). Responses to depressed interpersonal behavior: Mixed reactions in a helping role. *Journal of Personality and Social Psychology, 52*, 1274-1282.

Stuart, R. B. (1980). *Helping couples change: A social learning approach to marital therapy*. New York: Guilford.

Taylor, D. (1979). Motivational bases. In G. Chelune (Ed.), *Self-disclosure: Origins, patterns, and implications of openness in interpersonal relationships*. San Francisco: Jossey-Bass.

Taylor, S. E., & Brown, J. D. (1988). Illusion and well-being: A social psychological perspective on mental health. *Psychological Bulletin, 103*, 193-210.

Tennant, C., Bebbington, P., & Hurry, J. (1981). The short-term outcome of neurotic disorders in the community: The relation of remission to clinical factors and to 'neutralizing' life events. *British Journal of Psychiatry, 139*, 213-220.

Thibaut, J. W., & Kelley, H. H. (1959). *The social psychology of groups*. New York: Wiley.

Thoits, P. A. (1986). Social support as coping assistance. *Journal of Consulting and Clinical Psychology, 54*, 416-423.

Thomssen, C., & Möller, H.-J. (1988). A description of behavioral patterns of coping with life events in suicidal patients. In H.-J. Möller, A. Schmidtke, & R. Welz (Eds.), *Current issues of suicidology*. New York: Springer-Verlag.

Tienari, P., Sorri, A., Lahti, I., Naarala, M., Wahlberg, K.-E., Pohjola, J., & Moring, J. (1985). Interaction of genetic and psychosocial factors in schizophrenia. *Acta Psychiatrica Scandinavica* (Suppl. 319), *71*, 19-30.

Toldstedt, B. E., & Stokes, J. P. (1984). Self-disclosure, intimacy, and the depenetration process. *Journal of Personality and Social Psychology, 46*, 84-90.

Turkewitz, H., & O'Leary, K. D. (1981). A comparative outcome study of behavioral marital therapy and communication therapy. *Journal of Marital and Family Therapy, 7*, 159-169.

Uhlenhuth, E. H., Balter, M. D., Lipman, R. S., & Haberman, S. J. (1977). Remembering life events. In J. Strauss, H. Babigian, & M. Roff (Eds.), *The origins and course of psychopathology*. New York: Plenum.

Uhlenhuth, E. H., Lipman, R. S., Balter, M. B., & Stern, M. (1974). Symptom intensity and life stress in the city. *Archives of General Psychiatry, 31*, 759-764.

Vaillant, G. E. (1988). The alcohol-dependent and drug-dependent person. In A. M. Nicholi (Ed.), *The new Harvard guide to psychiatry*. Cambridge, MA: Harvard University Press.

Vanfossen, B. E. (1986). Sex differences in depression: The role of spouse support. In S. E. Hobfall (Ed.), *Stress, social support, and women*. Washington, DC: Hemisphere.

Vaughn, C. E., & Leff, J. P. (1976). The influence of family and social factors on the course of psychiatric illness: A comparison of schizophrenic and depressed neurotic patients. *British Journal of Psychiatry, 129*, 125-137.

Vivian, D., Smith, D. A., & O'Leary, K. D. (1988, November). *Emotional expression at premarriage as a predictor of discord at 18 and 30 months post marriage*. Paper presented at the 22nd annual meeting of the Association for Advancement of Behavior Therapy, New York.

Waring, E. M. (1988). *Enhancing marital intimacy through facilitating cognitive self-disclosure.* New York: Brunner/Mazel.

Warren, N. T. (1976). Self-esteem and sources of cognitive bias in the evaluation of past peformance. *Journal of Consulting and Clinical Psychology, 44,* 966–975.

Weiner, B., & Litman-Adizes, T. (1980). An attributional expectancy-value analysis of learned helplessness and depression. In J. Garber & M. Seligman (Eds.), *Human helplessness: Theory and applications.* New York: Academic.

Weiss, R. L. (1978). The conceptualization of marriage from a behavioral perspective. In T. Paolino, Jr., & B. McCrady (Eds.), *Marriage and marital therapy: Psychoanalytic, behavioral, and systems theory perspectives.* New York: Brunner/Mazel.

Weiss, R. L., & Aved, B. M. (1978). Marital satisfaction and depression as predictors of physical health status. *Journal of Consulting and Clinical Psychology, 46,* 1379–1384.

Weiss, R. L., & Birchler, G. R. (1978). Adults with marital dysfunction. In M. Hersen & A. S. Bellack (Eds.), *Behavior therapy in the psychiatric setting.* Baltimore: Williams & Wilkins.

Weiss, R. L., & Cerreto, M. C. (1980). The Marital Status Inventory: Development of a measure of dissolution potential. *American Journal of Family Therapy, 8*(2), 80–85.

Weiss, R. L., & Heyman, R. E. (1990). Marital distress and therapy. In A. S. Bellack, M. Hersen, & A. Kazdin (Eds.), *International handbook of behavior modification* (2nd ed.). New York: Plenum.

Weiss, R. L., Hops, H., & Patterson, G. R. (1973). A framework for conceptualizing marital conflict: A technology for altering it, some data for evaluating it. In L. A. Hamerlynck, L. C. Handy, & E. J. Mash (Eds.), *Behavior change: Methodology, concepts, and practice.* Champaign, IL: Research Press.

Weiss, R. S. (1974). The provision of social relationships. In Z. Rubin (Ed.), *Doing unto others.* Englewood Cliffs, NJ: Prentice-Hall.

Weissman, A. N., & Beck, A. T. (1978, November). *Development and validation of the Dysfunctional Attitude Scale: A preliminary investigation.* Paper presented at the annual meeting of the American Educational Research Association, Toronto, Ontario, Canada.

Weissman, M. M. (1979). The psychological treatment of depression: Evidence for the efficacy of psychotherapy alone, in comparison with, and in combination with pharmacotherapy. *Archives of General Psychiatry, 36,* 1261–1269.

Weissman, M. M. (1985, November). *Psychiatric epidemiology and clinical psychiatry: The new dialogue.* Paper presented in acceptance of the 1985 Rema Lapouse Mental Health Epidemiology Award at the annual meeting of the American Public Health Association, Washington, DC.

Weissman, M. M. (1987). Advances in psychiatric epidemiology: Rates and risks for major depression. *American Journal of Public Health, 77,* 445–451.

Weissman, M. M. (1988, November). *Conjoint versus individual interpersonal psychotherapy for depressed patients with marital disputes.* Paper presented at the 22nd annual meeting of the Association for the Advancement of Behavior Therapy, New York.

Weissman, M. M., Gershon, E. S., Kidd, K. K., Prusoff, B. A., Leckman, J. F., Dibble, E., Hamovit, J., Thompson, W. D., Pauls, D. L., & Guroff, J. J. (1984). Psychiatric disorders in the relatives of probands with affective disorders: The Yale–NIMH collaborative study. *Archives of General Psychiatry, 41,* 13–21.

Weissman, M. M., Klerman, G. L., & Paykel, E. S. (1971). Clinical evaluation of hostility in depression. *American Journal of Psychiatry, 128,* 261–266.

Weissman, M. M., Klerman, G. L., Paykel, E. S., Prusoff, B. A., & Hanson, B. (1974).

Treatment effects on the social adjustment of depressed patients. *Archives of General Psychiatry, 30,* 771–778.

Welz, R. (1988). Life events, current social stressors, and risk of attempted suicide. In H.-J. Möller, A. Schmidtke, & R. Welz (Eds.), *Current issues of suicidology.* New York: Springer-Verlag.

Welz, R., Veiel, H. O., & Hafner, H. (1988). Social support and suicidal behavior. In H.-J. Möller, A. Schmidtke, & R. Welz (Eds.), *Current issues of suicidology.* New York: Springer-Verlag.

Wender, P. H., Kety, S. S., Rosenthal, D., Schulsinger, F., Ortmann, J., & Lunde, I. (1986). Psychiatric disorders in the biological and adoptive families of adopted individuals with affective disorders. *Archives of General Psychiatry, 43,* 923–929.

Whisman, M. A., Jacobson, N. S., Fruzzetti, A. E.,. & Schmaling, K. B. (1988, November). *Treating the couple versus the depressed spouse alone: The short and long-term effects of cognitive behavior therapies for depression.* Paper presented at the 22nd annual meeting of the Association for Advancement of Behavior Therapy, New York.

Wicklund, R. (1975). Objective self-awareness. In L. Berkowitz (Ed.), *Advances in experimental social psychology* (Vol. 8). New York: Academic.

Wills, T. A., Weiss, R. L., & Patterson, G. R. (1974). A behavioral analysis of the determinants of marital satisfaction. *Journal of Consulting and Clinical Psychology, 42,* 802–811.

Wilson, G. T., O'Leary, K. D., & Nathan, P. N. (in press). *Abnormal psychology.* Englewood Cliffs, NJ: Prentice-Hall.

Winer, D. L., Bonner, T. O., Blaney, P. H., & Murray, E. J. (1981). Depression and social attraction. *Motivation and Emotion, 5,* 153–166.

Winokur, G. B., Clayton, P., & Reich, T. (1969). *Manic depressive illness.* St. Louis: Mosby.

Wortman, C. B. (1984). Social support and the cancer patient. *Cancer, 53,* 2339–2360.

Young, C. E., Giles, D. E., Jr., & Plantz, M. C. (1982). Natural networks: Help-giving and help-seeking in two rural communities. *American Journal of Community Psychology, 10,* 457–469.

Zilbergeld, B. (1978). *Male sexuality.* New York: Bantam.

# Index